10 Minutes to

Better Health

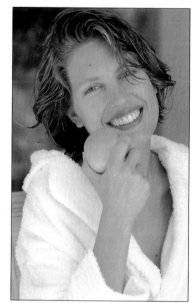

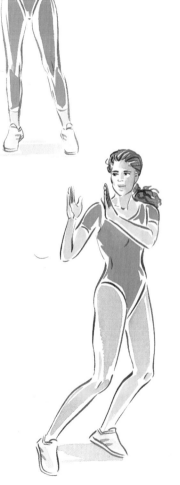

Jane Collins

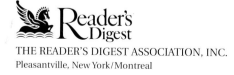

Reader's Digest

THE READER'S DIGEST ASSOCIATION, INC.

Pleasantville, New York/Montreal

A READER'S DIGEST BOOK

Produced by Tucker Slingsby Ltd

Copyright © 1999 Tucker Slingsby Ltd

Library of Congress Cataloging in Publication Data

Collins, Jane.
        10 minutes to better health: fast, effective ways
    to a fitter, more radiant you / Jane Collins.
            p.   cm.
    Includes index.
    ISBN 0-7621-0039-7
        1. Women—Health and hygiene—Popular works.
    2. Exercise for women—Popular works. 3. Beauty,
    Personal—Popular works.
    I.Title
    RA776.5.C64   1999
    613'.04244—dc21   98-30639

Manufactured in China

Contents

Ten minutes 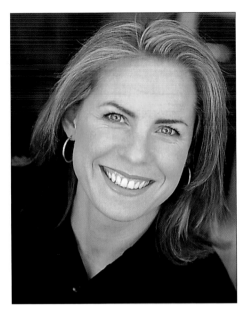 does make a difference!

All of us would like to be fitter, firmer, and have more zest for life. But finding time to exercise, eat well, look good, and practice relaxation techniques isn't easy! This book will show you how to use spare minutes to make a positive difference to your health. You won't need fancy exercise clothes; you won't need expensive equipment; and for most of the routines, you won't need to leave the house. All you really need is 10 minutes!

Prop open this specially designed, easy-to-use easel where you can't miss seeing it every day—on the kitchen counter, by the television,

or next to your bed. Open it to a page that interests you. As soon as you have 10 minutes to spare, try your chosen routine or recipe. If you enjoy it, incorporate it into your life; if not, try something else. There are over 200 exercises, relaxation routines, and beauty programs plus 100 healthy recipes to choose from. There are also hundreds of health tips and pages of invaluable information on how to get, and stay, healthy.

If you find it hard to get started, set the kitchen timer or an alarm clock to go off in 10 minutes. Tell yourself that when the buzzer sounds you

can stop your chosen routine. Remind yourself that 10 minutes isn't very long—just one percent of your waking day.

I guarantee that 10 minutes really can make a difference and set you on the path to a healthier, more enjoyable life. So take a little bit of time to look after yourself—you deserve it!

Jane Collins

BeforeYouBegin

Please take a few minutes to read this page before you begin any of the exercises or routines. All the information in this book has been written specially for busy women who have little time to keep fit, but if you haven't exercised at all for some time, or have any aches and pains, it is always best to consult a doctor before beginning an exercise program. Please note the special "Take Care" boxes that have been included to draw your attention to the health and safety aspects of specific routines and exercises.

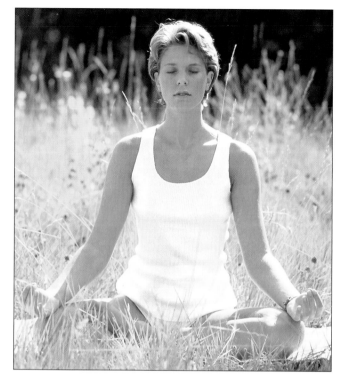

HOW TO USE THIS BOOK

This book is divided into five color-coded sections. Each of the sections addresses a different health or beauty concern. Look through the book to find the information that particularly applies to you. The unique easel design means you can leave your favorite page open, ready to use or refer to. Check out pages 124 and 125 at the back of the book—they will help you find 10-minute solutions to your problems at a glance.

SECTION 1—GetMoving!
Aerobic exercise gets your heart beating faster and your lungs working. It will increase your energy levels and make you feel great. Even if you haven't exercised for a while, this section is guaranteed to get you moving!

SECTION 2—Stretch&Tone
A fit, firm, flexible body can be yours—just take it 10 minutes at a time. There are exercises here to stretch and tone you from head to toe.

SECTION 3—EatWell
Fast food doesn't have to be unhealthy food. This section gives recipes for juices, breakfasts, snacks, packed lunches, soups, and main meals that are packed with goodness, and can be prepared in a matter of minutes.

SECTION 4—Calm&Relax
You can relax and de-stress yourself in minutes if you know the right techniques. There are relaxation and calming routines here to use at home, in the office, while traveling, and even while standing in line at the supermarket.

SECTION 5—LookGood
Time for skin, face, and hair care is usually the first casualty of a stressful lifestyle. Discover how 10-minute treatments can really improve your looks.

HealthTips
You'll find more clever ideas on how to maximize your exercise program, look great, save time, get organized, and realize your full, healthy potential in the Health Tips panels that are featured throughout the book. There are over 250 useful tips to try.

Clothes and shoes

The diagrams show women wearing leotards and leggings—this is to show the movements clearly. You don't need to wear special clothes. Do choose something comfortable—a tracksuit or T-shirt and shorts is fine. Try to change into your exercise gear as soon as you come home from work. Then you can grab any 10-minute opportunity that comes your way. Invest in some good exercise shoes. You will need to wear them for the stamina building (aerobic) exercises or when using weights (in case you drop them on your feet!). The right shoes make exercise a pleasure, not a chore.

1

GetMoving!

Why**Exercise?**

Exercise that gets your heart beating faster and develops your lung capacity—aerobic exercise—gives you energy and zest for life, helps you to maintain a healthy body weight, and can be great fun! You can begin simply by taking a brisk 10-minute walk every day. Then try some of the routines and exercises in this section. Take things slowly at first and build up your stamina, endurance, and energy levels gradually. You'll soon notice the difference.

EXERCISE

f you usually feel fatigued and never seem to get enough sleep, the last thing you probably feel like doing is exercising. Indeed, you may feel that an exercise routine will use up what little bit of spare energy you have—but really the complete opposite is true. Regular aerobic exercise will give you lots more energy and reduce the need for sleep. You will wake up feeling fresher and have more stamina to cope with everything the day throws at you.

Most of us don't want to run marathons or climb mountains—we just want to be fit enough to cope with working, playing with the kids, shopping, doing the chores—and have some energy left over to enjoy ourselves. This section offers realistic ideas for aerobic exercise that you can fit into a busy lifestyle. To begin with, concentrate on getting moving, even if it is only for a few minutes a day. Leave this book standing open at page 8 or page 9 and read the motivators when you need a push to get going.

When you rush in from the office or from taking the kids to school, try to resist the temptation to sit down with a cup of coffee.

ZEST

Have an energy-boosting banana, put on your favorite music track, and take 10 minutes to get moving with the aerobic exercise ideas on the following pages. You'll be surprised how quickly the minutes tick by and how much you enjoy yourself. Set the kitchen timer or an alarm clock if you need to

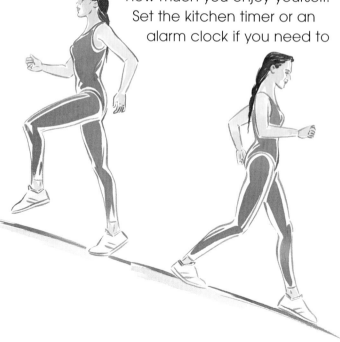

HEALTH

know when 10 minutes is up. If you still have energy, go on to one of the other 10-minute routines, or turn to Section 2—Stretch & Tone for exercises to improve your flexibility.

You'll find 10 minutes of exercise makes you feel more energetic physically, mentally, and emotionally. Keep up the effort and you'll soon be looking at a strong, new you!

Take Care

- **If you are pregnant, are on any medication, or suffer from any illness, consult your doctor before you begin. Take things easy and build your exercise routines up gradually, particularly if you haven't done any exercise for a while.**
- **It is normal for your heart to beat faster and for you to become breathless and sweat during sustained aerobic exercise. Stop immediately, however, if you feel nauseous, dizzy, light-headed, experience severe breathlessness, chest pain, pain in neck and arms, or heart palpitations.**
- **If after taking regular exercise and making other changes to your lifestyle, you still feel chronically tired, consult a doctor.**

Getting Started

I f you think that exercise is not for you, think again; the benefits you will gain from just a small amount of physical activity will far outweigh the effort.

TEN REASONS FOR EXERCISING

1 You will look better
Exercise will make you look firmer, slimmer, and better, both in and out of your clothes. Exercise improves posture, too.

2 You will be happier
Doing vigorous exercise for at least 10 minutes will help to trigger the production of endorphins, which are your body's feel-good chemicals.

3 You will burn up calories
Exercising will help you lose weight and keep you at your ideal weight. Just a few 10-minute blocks of continuous exercise, including brisk walking, running upstairs, swimming, even strenuous housework or gardening, will get your heart pumping faster. This will increase your metabolic rate and help you burn fat faster, even when you've stopped exercising.

4 You will suffer less from stress
Getting active will help you relax. A 10-minute walk can help to reduce stress, tension, and stress-related problems such as headaches and insomnia.

5 You will have more resistance to illnesses
Aerobic exercise reduces the risk of heart disease, bowel disease, diabetes, strokes, and osteoporosis. Exercise boosts the immune system and helps you to fight off colds and flu.

6 You will have more energy
Getting moving increases energy levels. Ask your friends how they are and you can guarantee someone will answer wearily: "Exhausted," or "I feel I could sleep for a week." Fatigue is one of the most common symptoms heard by medical practitioners. Although you can't get rid of fatigue completely—it's natural to feel tired when you're doing a lot—you'll notice an improvement in your energy levels in as little as one week if you take regular exercise. After three months you should have improved your strength considerably.

7 You will have great skin
Exercise makes your skin glow because it improves your circulation. Exercise improves the appearance of cellulite, too.

8 You will feel more confident
Being fit boosts your self-esteem. Looking better, feeling stronger, having more energy and enthusiasm, being more able to deal with stress—all these benefits of exercise will make you feel more confident.

9 You will feel more alert
Exercise makes you mentally fitter. It increases the supply of oxygen and glucose to the brain, which helps improve your concentration.

10 You will be helping family and friends
Increasing your fitness can improve the health of your family and friends. Encourage them to exercise with you or make exercise a social event that you enjoy together. Exercising with a friend or partner or with the whole family is a great motivator. If one of you feels too tired to bother—the other can usually provide support and encouragement.

Take Care

Try this simple test to assess how fit you are now, before you start on your new path to health and fitness. Do 5 minutes of continuous exercise such as fast walking or slow jogging. If you are gasping for breath and unable to speak you are doing too much, need to slow down, and are probably not very fit. If you are able to hold a conversation quite normally, you're not pushing yourself enough and can work a bit harder. Do this "talk test" again 6–8 weeks after starting your exercise routine. You will be impressed with the improvement.

Get Motivated

Don't agonize over exercise—just do it! The few minutes wasted wondering whether or not you have the time or energy for a walk can usefully be spent running in place. Leave this page open somewhere you will see it every day and use these motivators to help yourself get moving.

TEN MARVELOUS MOTIVATORS

1 It's okay to goof sometimes
Don't feel a failure if you have a bad health day—simply start again the following day. Don't set unrealistic goals and overdo exercise, or you will risk injuring yourself. You'll also get disheartened if you set yourself a pace you can't maintain. The key is patience and perseverance—inch your way into fitness with just 10 minutes of activity a day.

2 You don't have to leave the house
If you feel reluctant to walk around the streets or to attend an exercise class, exercise at home. Choose a time when no one is around to comment on your shape or size. When you have gained enough confidence to go to a class, you'll find people there look at themselves much more than they look at you!

3 Give yourself aromatherapy treats
Inhale stimulating aromatherapy essential oils such as lemon, tangerine, mandarin, rosemary, or basil to help lift feelings of lethargy and fatigue. Apply the oils to a tissue and inhale to pep yourself up before taking a short brisk walk or doing 10-minute bursts of aerobic exercise.

4 Always eat well
The most common reasons for an energy low are either a lack of food or the consumption of too much sugary junk food. Eat regular meals that include plenty of starchy carbohydrates. Snack on small amounts of carbohydrate, such as rice cakes, or fresh vegetables and fruit instead of chocolate bars or pastries. Graze instead of bingeing.

5 Use your imagination
Picture yourself with the toned, taut body you would like to have. As you do exercises for different parts of your body, imagine how you want that part of your body to look. See the muscles tightening and firming. Imagine yourself bursting with energy.

6 Don't worry about weight
Muscle weighs more than fat, so don't get disheartened if you are doing fat-busting exercises but not losing weight. You may be replacing "fat weight" with "muscle weight." It's better to judge your progress by the fit of your clothes.

7 Sleep well
Try to go to bed and get up at roughly the same time each day. Aim for at least seven hours' sleep. Get up when you wake up, even if you feel tired. Do some wake-up stretches. Research has shown that those who take regular exercise get a better night's sleep—so exercise will mean you wake up energetic, not lethargic.

8 Try something new
Vary the exercise you do. Nothing creates apathy more than boredom. If you can't bring yourself to exercise because you're fed up with doing the same activity, you simply won't do it. Try something different—such as rollerblading, rowing, swimming, or bicycling—when you feel bored with the exercise routines you normally do.

9 Make exercise a habit
Experts say you have to do something every day for a month for it to develop into a habit. Plan exercise into your routine—write it in your schedule—and don't let anyone steal that time.

10 Give me more!
You'll soon get to the stage when you miss exercise if you don't do it. That's when you'll know you are truly motivated!

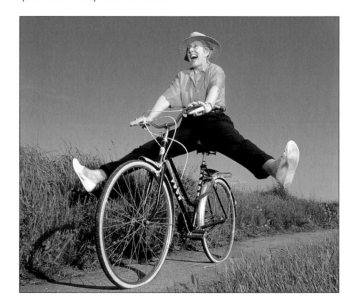

House Workout

You probably exercise for at least 10 minutes a day already! Housework and gardening shape up your body by toning muscles and improving flexibility. Put a bit more effort into sweeping, vacuuming, digging, or car-cleaning to give your heart and lungs a great workout.

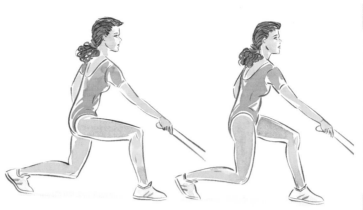

TEN CALORIE-BURNING TIPS

1 Wash up and tone your buttocks
Ten minutes' washing dishes burns 25 calories. Tone your behind at the same time by clenching your buttocks, squeezing, and holding for a couple of seconds, then releasing. Do this every time you stand at the kitchen sink and your buttocks should soon be firmer.

2 Iron and tone your legs
Ten minutes of ironing burns up around 25 calories. Increase the calories you burn, and tone up your legs by clenching and unclenching your abdomen and thigh muscles as you iron.

3 Shop and burn calories
You can burn up around 40 calories doing 10 minutes' shopping and around another 60 calories if you take a 10-minute brisk walk to get to the store—and the same again if you walk back.

4 Vacuum and lunge
Ten minutes' vacuuming will burn up 35 calories; increase the number of calories, and tone up your legs and buttocks, by doing lunges as you push the vacuum cleaner. Hold onto the vacuum with one hand. Lunge forward with your right leg keeping your left leg behind you, lowering your left knee toward the floor. Return to standing position. Continue to lunge forward, alternating your legs.

5 Run, don't walk, up the stairs
Increase your energy levels, your stamina, and the number of calories you burn by running up and down the stairs as often as you can. Take the stairs two at a time to work out your rear end.

6 Backpack bonus
Use a backpack to carry your shopping. This will improve stamina and strength because it allows you to swing your arms and work your upper body (see Power Walking on page 19) as you walk. Make sure the weight is evenly balanced and never carry it swung over one shoulder.

7 Clean the car and tone your upper body
Cleaning the car for 10 minutes will burn up around 45 calories, but you can increase the fat-burning potential by intensifying your arm action. Work out your arms and chest by using large, sweeping, circular movements as you wash and polish. When polishing a table, make wide circular motions using both arms, and press hard into the surface. This will help to strengthen and tone your chest and arm muscles.

8 Dust and stretch
Dusting burns up 25 calories in 10 minutes, but you can adapt it to work in some stretches plus arm toning and strengthening. Use a feather duster to skim around the ceiling corners. Stretch your arm high and bend slightly to one side. Hold for 10–20 seconds. Then work the other side of your body.

9 Mow the lawn and build stamina
Gardening is good for you—10 minutes' weeding burns 35 calories. Mowing the lawn burns up to 50 calories in 20 minutes. Mowing uphill burns another 25 calories, builds stamina, and provides a resistance weight for toning up your arms.

10 Snack and stay slim
One hour's hard housework burns off 250 calories—the same as bicycling for 30 minutes. When you have finished, reward yourself with a tasty 10-minute snack from Section 3—Eat Well. Resist the temptation to sit down with a donut!

EnergyDip Workout

Try this easy routine any time during the day when you have an energy dip. It's a great way to energize yourself if you wake up tired. Inspired by Eastern exercise therapies, these moves flood the body with revitalizing oxygen and make you feel more awake and alert. The routine also increases flexibility. If you have time, follow this 5-minute workout with 5 minutes' slow jogging or marching in place, or continue with the stretches on page 12.

THE RAGDOLL

1 Stand with your feet shoulder-width apart, bend your knees slightly, and let your upper body hang limply down toward the floor. Feel your back lengthen.

2 Breathe in and slowly curl your upper body up, keeping your knees bent and using your thigh muscles (not your back) to lift yourself. As you rise to hip level, cross your arms and continue slowly curling upward.

3 When your arms reach shoulder level, uncross them. Breathe out forcefully as you extend your arms upward. Repeat the exercise 3–5 times, inhaling deeply before you start each repetition, so you create a continuous, invigorating motion.

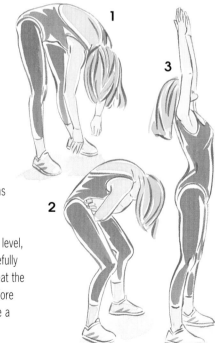

REACH UP TO THE CEILING

1 This stretching exercise relieves stress and stretches the area around the ribs, spine, and stomach muscles. Stand with your feet apart, knees slightly bent. Check your shoulders are relaxed. Breathe in slowly.

2 Breathe out slowly while you reach up with your right arm, palm pointing toward the ceiling. Stretch through the wrist so your hand flexes. Hold for 10 seconds as you breathe in, exhale, and stretch the left arm up as you lower the right. Repeat 3 times on each side.

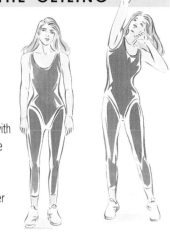

HIP ROTATIONS

1 Stand with feet a little more than shoulder-width apart, bend your knees, and move your arms in front of your chest with elbows bent as if you are holding a ball. Inhale deeply, relaxing your neck and shoulders, and imagine your breath filling your torso down to the base of your spine.

2 Breathe out slowly, and gently rotate your hips in a clockwise direction, stretching your hips as far as you can. Move your arms around in front in time with your hips. Repeat counter-clockwise. Make 10–12 circles in alternate directions.

HELPFUL HEALTH TIPS

■ You can use this routine prior to energetic exercise instead of the warm-up sequence on page 12. The Ragdoll movement is particularly effective as a warm-up since it focuses on loosening up your lower back.

■ Don't leave your workout until too late in the day, since this may make it difficult for you to sleep. If your only chance to exercise is late in the evening, turn to the stretches in Section 4—Calm & Relax.

■ Eating the right foods regularly will help boost your energy levels, too. An energy slump after a large lunch is almost inevitable. Check out the packed lunches, light meals, and snacks in Section 3—Eat Well.

WarmingUp

Before doing any sort of strenuous activity, whether it's power walking or a game of tennis, you should warm up and stretch to increase the blood flow to your muscles. Even the super fit risk injury if they suddenly force their muscles to work hard without warming up first. Do this warm-up sequence as a mini-workout in its own right or do it for 5 minutes before moving onto another routine.

Golden Rules of Exercise

- Do wear loose, comfortable clothes and a good sports bra.
- Do invest in proper aerobic training shoes. Don't do aerobic exercise or use weights in bare feet.
- Do have a light snack, such as a small banana or a glass of fruit juice, before exercising in the evening if you haven't eaten since lunch. Don't exercise for at least an hour after a meal.
- Do take notice of injuries. Don't exercise if you feel any twinges of pain.
- Do take things at your own pace and don't overtrain.
- Do have water to drink when exercising.

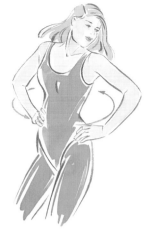

1 Circle your hips as if you are swinging a hoop around. Do 30 seconds clockwise, then 30 seconds counter-clockwise.

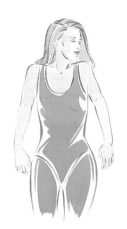

2 Stand with feet hip-width apart. Circle your shoulders forward for 30 seconds, then backward for 30 seconds.

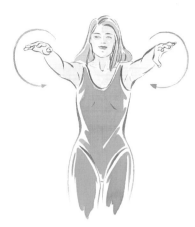

3 Hold your arms out in front of you. Circle inward with both arms, 5 times, then repeat, circling outward 5 times.

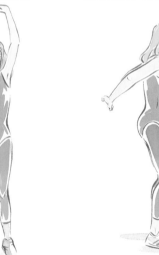

4 Stand with feet hip-width apart. Lift your arms above your head and link fingers with your palms pointing toward the ceiling. Stretch and hold for 20 seconds.

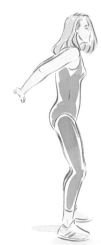

5 Clasp your hands behind your back with your palms facing downward and slowly move your arms up. Hold the stretch for a count of 5 and repeat.

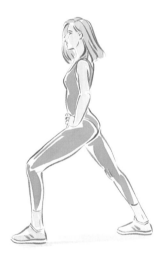

6 Take a big step forward with your left leg, so it is bent at the knee and the heel of your right leg is flat on the floor. Hold for 5–10 seconds then change legs.

HELPFUL HEALTH TIPS

■ Warm up immediately before an exercise routine. If you leave more than 10 minutes between doing your warm-up and starting to exercise, your body will cool down again.

■ Mentally focus on the muscles you are working when you stretch in steps 4, 5, and 6. This will make the movements much more effective. Breathe deeply and evenly throughout the warm-up to help you relax and concentrate.

■ There are lotions and sprays to relieve muscle pain and stiffness following exercise. These should never be used as a substitute for warming up—they do not help to prevent injuries, but a warm-up will.

■ Stretch out after exercise with the Cooling Down exercises on page 23—stopping exercise abruptly can be as dangerous as starting without a warm-up.

StepsToFitness

You don't need to use a step machine to enjoy the health benefits of a step aerobics class. Running up stairs for 10 minutes can burn off 350 calories and even walking up them for the same amount of time can burn off around 150. You can also use your stairs at home to do stationary exercises. You will need a staircase (or a store-bought step), and tin cans or bottles of water to use as weights. Do the warm-up on page 12 before you begin.

BASIC STEPPING

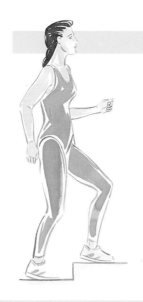

Walk up and down your stairs three times, trying to increase your speed if you can. Rest for a few minutes. Step on and off the bottom stair. Lead with the same foot for a couple of minutes—right foot up, left foot up, right foot down, left foot down, then change the leading foot. Repeat this exercise for up to 10 minutes.

Do the warm-up on page 12 before you begin.

STEPPING FORWARD

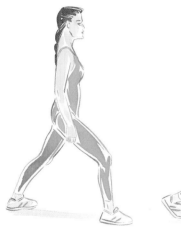
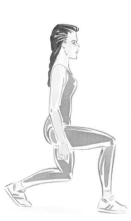
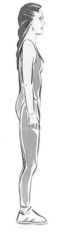
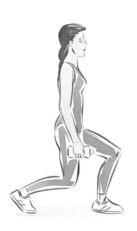

1 Stand with arms by your sides. Step forward onto your right leg as if you are about to stride forward. Keep your left leg behind you and body erect.

2 Bend your right leg, then bend your left leg toward the floor. Let your heel come up. Aim to get your left knee about 4 in (10 cm) off the floor.

3 Slowly go back to the starting position and change legs. Continue for up to 5 minutes, increasing to 10 minutes after a few weeks.

4 When you feel comfortable doing these exercises, try holding a couple of tin cans or plastic water bottles down by your sides as you do them.

KNEE LIFT

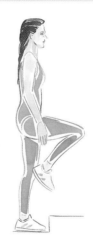

Step up on a stair with your left leg, lift your right knee up, step down with your right foot, then your left. Repeat, alternating the leading foot, for 5 minutes.

HELPFUL HEALTH TIPS

■ When walking up and down the stairs, or doing the step exercises opposite, try to pump your arms—the rhythm will come naturally—to give you a total body workout. This will help work your heart, lungs, and muscles, and improve circulation.

■ If you enjoy stepping, try a class. The instructor will be able to teach you choreographed moves to work out your arms and legs to achieve total fitness.

Take Care

It's important to monitor your heart rate during and just after aerobic exercise to make sure you are working within safe limits and maximize the fat-burning capacity of exercise. First, calculate your maximal heart rate by subtracting your age from 220. For example, a 40-year-old's top heart rate should be 180 beats per minute. Beginners should work at about 60 percent of this rate—108 beats per minute. As you get fitter, this can increase to 70 percent, working up to 85 percent (153 beats per minute).

Start-up Moves

These exercises are an excellent way to start developing a stamina-building routine. Try to spend a couple of minutes doing each of the moves. Increase the intensity of the exercises by adding larger swinging or punching arm movements or by making the leg movements bigger or faster. Stretch out for a few minutes before beginning (see page 12). Leave yourself a minute or two to cool down at the end.

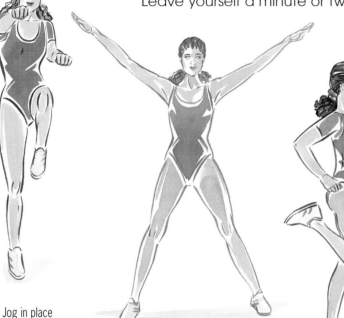

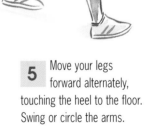

1 March in place, building up speed gradually. Lift your knees up high and swing alternate arms, as if you were running, to give yourself a full body workout.

2 Jog in place while "punching" alternate arms straight out in front of you.

3 Do jumping jacks for 2 minutes. Stand with legs together and arms down by your sides. Jump so that your legs are apart and your arms are above your head and your body forms an "X" shape. Jump back, bringing your legs together and your arms back to your sides.

4 Bring your right heel up to your right buttock, then the left heel up to the left buttock. Keep alternating this heel-to-buttock movement as quickly as you can.

5 Move your legs forward alternately, touching the heel to the floor. Swing or circle the arms.

■ If you are new to exercise, you may find even a few minutes tough going. Try to persevere. Imagine you have a personal trainer in the room and he or she is making you do an extra minute of each exercise. You'll get a surge of energy after 5 minutes of exercise. This is when the brain releases chemicals called endorphins into the body. These give you a natural high.

■ Exercising to upbeat music can help to sustain you for longer and is fun, so you tend to forget you are exercising. Try these exercises to your favorite tunes.

Take Care

To prevent injury during aerobic activity, warm up for a few minutes before starting and stretch out afterward (see pages 12 and 23). Avoid locking, or completely straightening, your knees and elbows during any exercise to minimize stress to ligaments. Make sure you do not work out on your toes—place your whole foot down toe to heel during aerobic movements.

BurnFatFaster

To lose fat from your body, you need to increase your heart rate and work hard enough to get out of breath. Try this fat-burning routine when you have 10 minutes to spare. March in place for 2 minutes to warm up, lifting your knees high.

1 Kick alternate legs out in front and punch forward alternate arms. Keep the movements smooth to maintain momentum. Continue for 1 minute.

2 Lift alternate feet, touching your buttocks with your heel. As you lift, bend your arms at the elbows and make fists with your hands, bringing them up to your shoulders. Continue for 1 minute.

3 Jog as fast as you can in place for 30 seconds to 1 minute.

4 Briskly walk up and down a flight of stairs. Gain speed as you go up and come down at a controlled pace. Continue for 2 minutes.

5 Stand upright, stomach pulled in, feet together, and arms in front of thighs. Kick alternate legs out to the side, raising them 4 in (10 cm); swing arms to shoulder level. Continue for 2 minutes.

6 Step to the right. Bring your left foot in and tap it against the right. Step to the left and tap the right foot against the left. Take 2–4 steps in one direction before going back the other way. Continue for 1 minute.

7 Cool down for a couple of minutes by walking in place and gently shaking out your arms and legs.

HELPFUL HEALTH TIPS

■ Regular exercise is the key to fitness. It's much better for your stamina and your muscles to do 10 minutes of exercise a day, than one hour once a week.

■ Match your calorie intake to your level of activity. On your "rest days," when you are not doing fat-burning exercise, focus on eating fresh fruit and salad. On very active days, you will need to eat more carbohydrates, such as pasta and rice.

■ You cannot selectively burn off fat, so no matter how many sit-ups you do, for example, you will not reduce the fat, or cellulite, from your stomach simply by concentrating all your efforts on it. The key is to mix aerobic work with targeted sculpting exercises to burn up fat and tone specific areas of your body (see Section 2—Stretch & Tone.)

Dance Moves

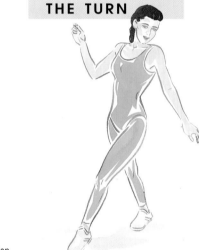

Dance-style steps are perfect to get you moving, increase your heart rate, and get your lungs working. Create your own 10-minute workout by putting on your favorite music and making up a routine from the steps shown here, plus any of the steps on pages 14 and 15, alternating them with jogging or marching in place. Start gently to give your muscles a chance to warm up, and slow down gradually.

THE GRAPEVINE

1 The grapevine is a simple step to start with. It's used as a basic element of most aerobic class routines. Stand with your feet together. Step to the left side, leading with your left foot.

2 Your right foot follows, stepping behind your left foot, so that your feet are crossed. You can work harder by using your arms during the movement. Swing them out to the side as you cross your feet and bring them in as you step again.

3 Step left again with your left leg, the right foot follows and you step together. Keep thinking: "Step wide, cross behind, step wide, step together." Repeat the grapevine steps (1–3) to the right.

THE MAMBO

This is a Latin-style step. With your feet together, step forward diagonally with your right leg crossing your left. Allow your right hip to sway forward, Latin-style, transferring your weight onto your front foot. Step your right foot back, allowing your hip to sway back, and bring your feet together. Repeat on the other side.

THE TURN

This move is called the pivot turn. With feet together, keep your right foot on the spot and step your left foot forward and around, turning your body to the right, pivoting on the ball of your right foot. Take three steps to turn around until you are facing forward again.

■ For these dance exercises, make sure you have enough space to move at least four steps forward, backward, and side to side.

■ Time your 10 minutes by selecting your favorite CD tracks of upbeat, motivating music.

■ Moderate dancing burns around 7 calories per minute, but vigorous dancing burns 100 calories in 10 minutes.

■ If you enjoy strutting your stuff, why not learn some professional moves, either by attending a class or watching an instruction video? You'll find a huge variety of styles on offer, which suit different levels of fitness and musical tastes. Look out for classes in jazz, Irish dancing, salsa, line dancing, and ballroom dancing.

MachineWorkout

Most of us have, at some time, invested in home exercise equipment—probably inspired by a model on an info-mercial. What usually happens is that the machine gets used intensively for a few weeks, then less and less frequently. Eventually it gets packed up and sits in a closet collecting dust. Now is the time to get the machine back into action. If you don't have one, shop around to find a machine that suits your budget and interest. Or check with your friends—someone may well have an unused machine. Swapping machines when you get bored is also a good idea. Ten minutes on your machine, whether it's a bicycle, ski machine, stepper, treadmill, or rowing machine, makes for a great workout. Fast walking or light bicycling both burn

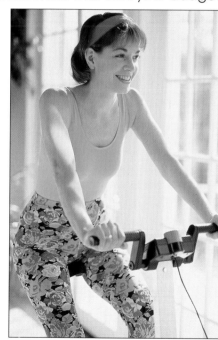

about 40 calories in 10 minutes. Bicycling hard, jogging, or running use 100 calories in 10 minutes.

TEN-MINUTE TREADMILL

1 Walk at a moderate to fast pace for 2 minutes to warm up. Move your arms in an exaggerated way so you are getting a total body workout.

2 Continue at the same pace, but switch the machine to an uphill level for 2 minutes so you are walking on an uphill incline. Keep moving your arms.

3 Switch the machine back to the flat gradient and increase your pace so you break into a faster walk or slow run. Continue for 5 minutes.

4 Reduce your speed so you are walking at a moderate pace to help you cool down slowly for 1 minute.

TEN-MINUTE BICYCLE

1 Pedal slowly for 1 minute to warm up your muscles.

2 Increase your speed and bicycle for up to 5 minutes at a moderately fast pace.

3 Switch the bicycle machine to uphill and pedal for another 3 minutes.

4 Switch back to flat gradient and reduce your speed for the last minute to cool down slowly.

TEN-MINUTE ROW

1 Pull the handle in toward your stomach as you glide gently back and forth on the seat. Do this slowly for 2 minutes.

2 Increase the speed at which you "row" and pull the handle in toward your stomach as you move back and forth on the seat. Keep the motion smooth and strong, not jerky and uncoordinated. Continue for 5 minutes.

3 For 1 minute only, concentrate really hard on keeping your arm movements as strong and as fast as you can. Imagine you are in a boat race and are heading toward the finish line.

4 Gradually slow down your "rowing" speed for 2 minutes, but try not to lose momentum. Continue to keep your arm movements strong and smooth as you cool down slowly.

HELPFUL HEALTH TIPS

■ When buying or borrowing an exercise machine for home use or using one in the gym, make sure you understand exactly how it works. Get an expert to show you all the features and the correct techniques for using it. Injury can occur if your technique is bad or you don't understand how to increase or decrease the speed.

■ When buying machines, go to a reputable sporting goods store and test all the models. As a rule, it is probably better to go for something that is middle range in price—if it's too cheap, the machine can be flimsy and may not have additional features such as uphill work, heart-rate monitor, or a facility that counts the number of calories you have used up.

■ Always be aware of your limits when using machines. It can sometimes be good to push yourself a bit further, but never push yourself if you feel pain or feel dizzy or faint.

WalkYourselfFit

Walking is one form of exercise that most of us can easily incorporate into our lives. Slow walking burns about 4 calories per minute; brisk walking burns 7 calories per minute—so a 10-minute walk burns at least 40 calories. Walking also improves endurance, stamina, and overall fitness. Like other weight-bearing aerobic exercise, walking helps protect you from osteoporosis. It can also raise your spirits and help you to deal with stress and tension. A 10-minute walk raises energy levels for up to 2 hours—try going for a walk in your lunch break to prevent a mid-afternoon energy slump.

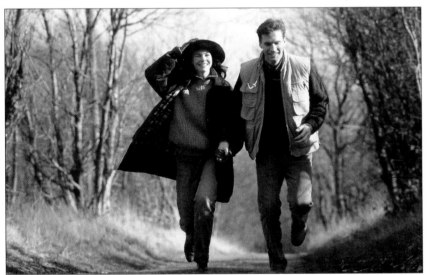

TEN WAYS TO GET WALKING

1 Walk part of the way
Start by walking part of the way to the store or to work. If you travel by bus, subway, or train, get off a stop early and walk. Go at a slow pace initially and build up speed and distance gradually.

2 Be a social walker
Incorporate walking into your social life. Instead of taking part in sedentary social activities such as going to the movies or a bar, organize walks on weekends and summer evenings. Eat a meal afterward, if you like. After a walk your body actually increases the rate at which it burns off calories—even after you've stopped exercising.

3 Pick up speed
Walk fast enough to become a little breathless and slightly tired, but do not leave yourself gasping for air or totally exhausted. Breathe deeply and evenly, taking plenty of fresh air into your lungs.

4 Relax
Keep your joints relaxed but not floppy. Avoid jarring your knees, hips, and back by making sure that your knees are slightly bent when your feet hit the ground. Try to walk on grass rather than concrete.

5 Start gradually
Start with a 10-minute walk a day and build up gradually. Work out a circular route that you can do in 10 minutes. Extend it as you get fitter. Vary your routes if you get bored. Aim to build up to walking 2 miles (3 km) at least three times a week. It isn't as far as it sounds—for an average adult this should take around 30 minutes.

6 Don't take the elevator
Walk up stairs instead of taking the elevator. Ten minutes' stair-climbing can burn off 150 calories.

7 Swing your arms
When you walk, use your arms to get a full workout. They should swing slightly in sync with your stride, but don't pump them back and forth, this will slow you down. Keep your arms swinging close to your body to keep you balanced.

8 Walk—don't run
Don't overstride or break into a run. Maintain your momentum and you'll walk farther and faster, without straining your joints or spine.

9 Get good shoes
Wear well-fitting, comfortable shoes when walking or you may damage your feet. Shop for walking shoes in the afternoon when your feet have expanded. Try to make sure there is a ¼ in (5 mm) space between your longest toe and the front of your shoe.

10 Walk to create more energy
Help your body create even more energy by increasing the intensity of your walk as your fitness improves. Work against resistance—by pushing a baby buggy uphill or against the wind. You'll increase your oxygen intake and feel even fitter.

Power Walking

ower walking is a fancy name for walking briskly—roughly a mile (1.5 km) in 12 minutes. By moving at this pace, you exercise all the major muscle groups without the high-impact action of jogging or running. Power walk anywhere and at any time for just 10 minutes to get your heart beating, help you burn fat, and improve general fitness. If you don't already walk regularly, check out the information on page 18 before you start to power walk.

BEFORE YOU SET OUT

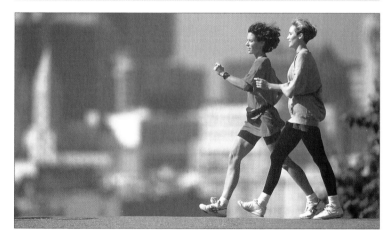

■ Eat a high-carbohydrate, energy-sustaining snack not less than an hour before you leave for your power walk. Foods such as rice, oatmeal, or pasta will help to keep you going. If you prefer, snack on a banana to give you a slow release of energy.

■ To avoid dehydration, drink plenty of water before, during, and after your walk. Carry water with you in a plastic bottle.

■ Do some warm-up stretches before you begin to power walk. The sequence on page 12 is a good guide. Cool down and stretch out after your walk.

HOW TO POWER WALK

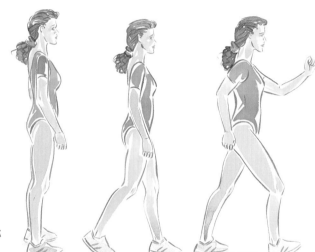

1 Lift your chest to make your back straight but not arched. Relax your shoulders, keep your head high and your chin up to help you breathe efficiently.

2 Pull your stomach in and lead from the chest. Take comfortable strides, but aim to increase their frequency—it is the speed of the walk, not the length of stride that helps to define leg muscles. Strike the ground with your heel first, then roll through to your toe.

3 Bend your arms at the elbow to form a 90-degree angle and let them swing as naturally as possible. Don't concentrate too hard on pumping your arms as this will slow you down.
Concentrate on what you're doing as you power walk. Feel your leg and buttock muscles contract, and your weight shift onto your heels. This helps you work harder and so burn up more calories.

HELPFUL HEALTH TIPS

■ Avoid power walking in areas of heavy congestion, especially if the air quality is poor. If you live in an area where the pollution levels are high, take an early morning walk when the air is at its cleanest.

■ Wear bright clothing and keep to well-lit, populated areas when out walking. Ideally go with a friend to help you feel more secure and motivated.

■ Wear a watch when you walk—preferably one with a stop-watch facility—so you can keep a check on your times. This will help you monitor your progress, too, which is great for motivation.

PuttingUp**AFight**

Boxing moves improve coordination, build up stamina, make your body stronger, and help you get rid of pent-up aggression. Do some warm-up marching and stretching before beginning (see page 12) and then do 10 minutes of brisk "boxercise." You will need a broom or stick for the lunge exercise.

SIDE KICKS

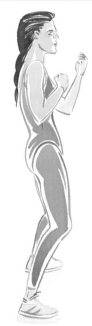 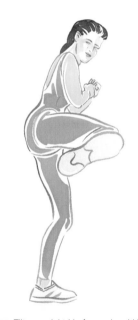

1 Stand with your knees slightly bent, hands held in fists, elbows bent, and hands up in front of your body at shoulder height.

2 Tilt your right hip forward and kick your right leg out to the side, leading with your buttock muscle. Keep foot flexed. Repeat 15 times. Switch legs.

PUNCHING

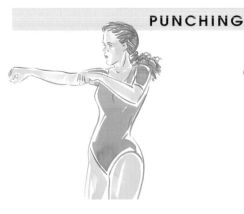 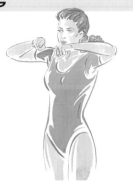

1 Make fists with your hands, backs of hands facing the ceiling, and punch your arms straight out in front of you. Continue for 2 minutes and relax.

2 Draw your fists up close to your face and make short punching movements in the air. Increase your speed. After 2 minutes repeat step 1.

LIFTING LUNGE

1 Lunge your right leg out in front, foot flat on the floor, making a 90-degree angle with your knee. The knee should not go beyond your ankle. Keep the left leg behind you, directly under hip. Slide a stick or broom handle under your right knee. Your back should be straight and your stomach held in tight.

2 Lift and lower the broom handle slowly from under your right knee to the floor 10 times—your left knee should try to touch the floor. Change legs and repeat for another 10. This exercise works the arms, thighs, and buttocks.

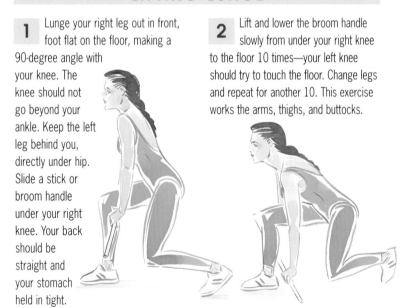

■ If you enjoy doing these boxing moves, you can learn more by watching a boxercise video or attending a class, where you can use a punchbag to get rid of all that pent-up aggression!

■ Jumping rope makes an excellent warm-up for boxing exercises and is a good aerobic activity, which is why so many professional boxers do it. You can extend this routine by jumping rope for 2 minutes at a jogging pace after your warm-up stretches and before you go into the boxing exercises.

■ Remember to drink plenty of water before, during, and after strenuous exercise. Put a bottle of water out ready before you begin an exercise routine. If you don't normally drink much water, you will be surprised to find how much you really appreciate it after exercise—and drinking more water is a great, healthy habit to get into.

Skipping**Fit**

Skipping builds energy levels and burns off fat quickly—10 calories a minute—the same as a professional playing basketball. Warm up with a few stretches (see page 12) before starting this 10-minute skipping routine. You will need aerobic shoes designed for high-impact exercise and a high-quality jump rope. The rope should be long enough to clear your head when you skip. If walking is your favorite form of exercise, you will find skipping a good substitute, especially when the weather is bad or you can't leave the house. It will remind you of games from your childhood, so it will make you smile too!

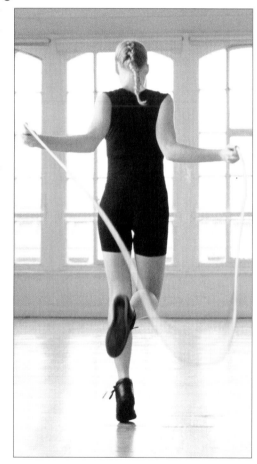

SKIP FOR STAMINA

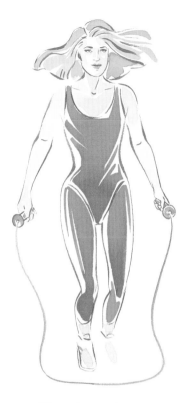
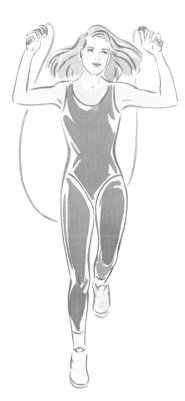

1 Skip continuously for 1 minute, hopping with alternate feet. Keep up a slow, comfortable pace.

2 Skip for 1 minute, keeping both feet together. Take an extra bouncing jump in between skips.

3 Skip at jogging pace with alternate feet for about 2 minutes, then take up to 1 minute's rest.

4 Do two 1-minute bursts at running speed, taking a 30-second rest in between. Use alternate feet not both feet together.

5 Do 2 minutes' skipping at a slower, jogging pace.

6 Cool down with a leisurely 1-minute skip.

HELPFUL HEALTH TIPS

■ Try to avoid skipping outdoors on concrete. It has the same jarring effect on your joints and muscles as jogging on the sidewalk. Far better to do it on a carpeted floor inside or on grass outside.

■ Skipping is high-intensity exercise and gets your heart pumping very quickly. If you find you can't manage 1 minute of continuous skipping to begin with, don't push yourself too hard. Try 30 seconds and build up slowly.

■ Shorten the jump rope by wrapping it around your hands to give yourself a harder workout.

■ Skipping will help to increase your stamina and make your body stronger. For complete all-round fitness, improve your flexibility with some of the stretches in Section 2—Stretch & Tone.

WaterWorkout

Exercising in water builds stamina, strength, and flexibility, and there is no danger of straining joints because the water bears your weight. The pressure of the water also provides resistance and makes your muscles work harder. Use this 10-minute underwater exercise sequence as a warm-up prior to swimming laps, or do the routine on its own.

WALKING THROUGH WATER

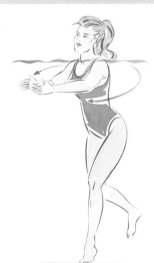 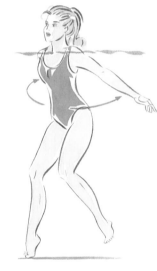

In water up to your shoulders, walk as fast as you can, pushing your arms forward and around in large sweeping movements under water. This is excellent for burning off fat and providing good all-over conditioning. Your legs get a good workout because they have to work against the force of the water; your stomach muscles are used more than if you were walking on land; and the upper back muscles and the pectoral muscles also get exercised. Continue for 2 minutes, building up to more.

LEG LIFTS

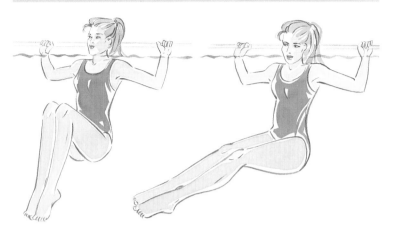

With your back pressed against the side of the pool, hold onto the edge as you lift and lower your legs, keeping them bent at the knees. Continue for 2–3 minutes. This will work the muscles at the front of the hip as well as the buttock muscles (gluteals). Bend, then straighten your legs out in front of you without lowering them to work the fronts and backs of your thighs. Continue for 2–3 minutes.

RUN IN DEEP WATER

Make running or cycling movements underwater using your hands to keep you afloat. If you are not a confident swimmer, you might feel more comfortable wearing a light life jacket to keep you afloat. Try to run from one side of the pool to the other. This works all the muscles in your legs and arms, and keeps your heart and lungs in good working order. It also quickly burns up calories. Try doing this for 2 minutes and build up to more as your stamina increases.

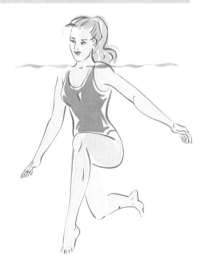

Cooling Down

Take time to stretch your muscles after all strenuous aerobic exercise. This will protect you from cramps and help reduce muscle stiffness. Stretching work done while your muscles are warm has the double benefit of cooling you down and helping you to keep flexible. You can also use these stretches at the end of a busy day to de-stress yourself.

FLEXIBILITY STRETCH

1 Lie on your back with your stomach pulled in and lower back pressed into the floor. Bend your right leg, keeping your right foot on the floor. Raise your left leg, sole toward the ceiling.

2 Clasp your left leg with both hands around the thigh or calf and gently pull your leg toward you. Stop when you feel the stretch, and before feeling any strain. Hold for 10–20 seconds. Relax and repeat both steps on the right leg.

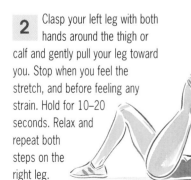

SHAKE OUT

1 If you have been running, power walking, skipping, or doing any other kind of intense aerobic exercise, slow down gradually, keeping going at a leisurely pace for a few minutes and gradually coming to a complete stop.

2 Shake your arms and legs out to help prevent stiffness and help you cool down.

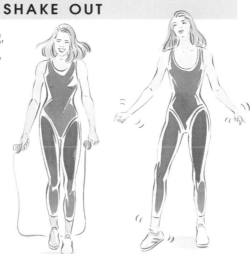

LEG STRETCHES

1 Take a big stride forward with your left foot. Check your hips are facing forward and feet are flat on the floor. The left leg should be slightly bent. Hold the stretch for a count of 20. Repeat on the right leg.

2 Bring the right leg forward, so it's straight in front of you, with the foot flexed. Lean your weight onto the bent left leg. Hold for a count of 10, release, and repeat on the other side.

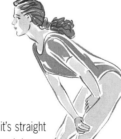

3 Stand upright (near a wall if you need support) and bring your left heel back toward your left buttock. Bend your right knee slightly, tuck your rear under, and keep knees together. Feel the stretch in the front of your thighs. Hold for 10–20 seconds, relax, and release. Repeat on the right leg.

HELPFUL HEALTH TIPS

■ Don't suddenly stop if you get tired during aerobic exercise. This could make you feel faint. When you exercise, your heart rate increases and your muscles produce a pumping action to accommodate the increased blood flow and speed the return of blood to the heart. If you stop suddenly, this pumping action also stops and the rate of blood flow into the muscles remains fast. The result is a pooling of blood in the veins that can make you feel light-headed and dizzy. Even if you feel tired, try to continue the exercise at a slow speed for a couple of minutes or walk to cool down.

■ If you cramp as you are cooling down, slowly walk around until the spasm subsides.

■ If you have time, finish your cool down by relaxing for 10 minutes. Lie down and stretch out. Put your arms down by your sides and breathe deeply. Focus on relaxing your muscles, one by one. For more relaxation information see page 98.

MovingOn

Once you have been doing 10 minutes' exercise a day for 6–8 weeks, you will want to—and find you can—do more. To continue improving your fitness, you will need to build up to between three and five aerobic sessions per week, with each session lasting at least 30 minutes. You may want to join a class or gym, but remember there are lots of fun ways to exercise that don't tie you down to a regular time. Swimming, cycling, and walking can all be enjoyed at any time and fitted into a busy day.

MORE EXERCISE, BETTER HEALTH

1 Walk more
Increase the pace and distance you walk. Setting a brisk pace while you walk can burn off 150 calories in 30 minutes. If you live near, or are vacationing near, a beach, walk on the sand barefoot. It's harder work, so exercises you more.

2 Try jogging
When you can easily walk 2 miles (3 km) in 30 minutes, try alternating walking with jogging. Slow down to a walk if you become tired and then continue. Invest in good running shoes.

3 Head for the hills
Get out into the country and try hill walking. Walking uphill shapes your legs, particularly your

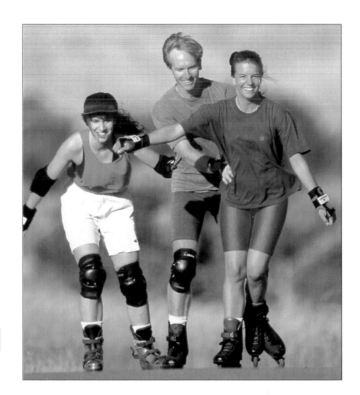

thighs and calves, as well as your buttocks. It also burns more calories than walking on the flat. Do not slump forward when you go uphill—carry your neck and spine straight, keep your shoulders pulled back and stomach tucked in. Control your strides going downhill and keep the same upright posture.

4 Swim yourself fitter
Go swimming more often to build stamina and endurance. Water is weight-bearing, so swimming is safe for pregnant women, the unfit, those with back or joint problems, and the elderly. Swim laps continuously for maximum benefit. Aim for 20 minutes, and build up to 40 minutes.

5 Enjoy a sport
Play a social sport, such as tennis, badminton, or squash. Most of these sports are played for 30–60 minutes. Try to play with people of the same experience and fitness level as you, so you don't push yourself too hard or lose motivation.

6 Work and play
Mix and match exercise routines and chores to fit 30 minutes of continuous activity into a busy schedule. For example, do 20 minutes' gardening, followed by 10 minutes' skipping.

7 Get a full body workout
Combine aerobic exercise with stretching and toning for a full body workout. Build up to these sessions gradually, just as you do with aerobic exercise (see Section 2—Stretch & Tone). Aim for two 30-minute toning sessions a week.

8 Join an aerobics class
Choose a class that suits your fitness level. Start with "low-impact" classes, which do not include jumping and jogging.

9 Try something new
Tackling new physical challenges will make you feel mentally stronger as well as fitter. Try roller-blading, ice skating, or horseback riding, which all give the lower body a good workout.

10 Get family and friends involved
Plan stamina-building fun activities you can enjoy with family and friends. Combine a walk in the park with rowing on the lake. Play catch or tag with the kids. Organize long walks in the country.

Stretch&Tone

UseItOrLoseIt!

No matter how unfit you feel, it will only take 10 minutes of gentle exercise a day to gain a more flexible body and a more youthful, sleeker shape. You'll feel more energetic and alive too. Getting fitter and firmer need not be difficult or time-consuming. It is simply a matter of working exercise into your day-to-day activities, so find 10 minutes to start toning up and getting flexible today!

Having a firm, taut body doesn't have to be solely the preserve of women in their teens and twenties. Developing stiff joints, slack muscles, back pain, knee pain, arthritic conditions, or weak bones are not

SHAPE

necessarily natural signs of aging. It is more likely that they are signs of a sedentary lifestyle, and unhealthy eating and drinking habits.

For a body that is more flexible and a shape that is sleeker, you don't have to pound the pavements or wear out the exercise bike. Start with 10 minutes of simple toning and stretching exercises to keep your body and your face looking younger. These exercises will help to prevent joint and bone problems, too. As you feel fitter and want

to do more, you can gradually build up to 20- and then 30-minute sessions by mixing and matching the exercises on the following pages.

Some of the routines concentrate on toning up particular problem areas including thighs, buttocks, stomach, and upper arms. Do a few minutes' warm-up before beginning any of these routines, to get your body used to moving and stretching.

The two reasons most of us give for not exercising more are—one: not having time and two: being too tired. Following 10-minute routines will really help you to overcome the disinclination to exercise. Tell yourself it is just for 10 minutes—then you can stop and sit down or get on with the rest of your busy day. You will soon find that exercising actually gives you energy and that you are looking forward to your 10-minute exercise break.

FLEXIBLE

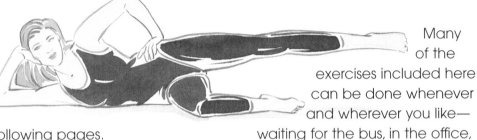

ENERGY

Many of the exercises included here can be done whenever and wherever you like— waiting for the bus, in the office, or at home. You can make instant exercise weights by filling plastic bottles with water, or by grabbing two tin cans from the kitchen.

Take Care

If you are pregnant, on medication, or suffer with back pain or any medical condition, consult your doctor before attempting the exercises in this book. Listen to your body—if you feel you are over-exerting yourself, or if any movement is uncomfortable, stop. Do not push yourself too far, especially if you are unfit and haven't exercised recently. Consult your physician if you have any reservations about your state of health. It's better to be cautious than rush into exercise and have to cope with injuries and related problems.

WakeUp WarmUp

This simple routine should be done before the start of any exercise routine to help warm up and stretch the muscles, so preventing the risk of injury.

GET READY, GET SET, GO

1 First warm up the lower back. Bend forward about 30 degrees, placing your hands above your kneecaps to support your back. Round out and then straighten your spine 8 times.

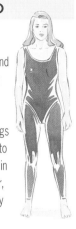

2 Warm up your whole body: stand tall and march gently in place for 1 minute. Increase the pace for 1 minute, lifting your legs higher. Step from side to side, bringing one foot in to tap against the other, for 1 minute. Jog gently in place for 1 minute.

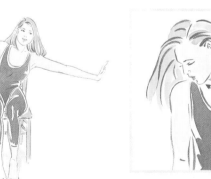

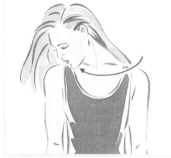

3 Stand with your feet apart or sit. Stretch your arms out and bend to the left to stretch your side. Hold for a count of 8, then repeat on the right side.

4 Drop your head onto your chest and slowly circle it to the left toward your shoulder. Circle back to the center, then to the right. Repeat 5 times.

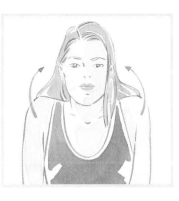

5 Shrug your shoulders up toward your ears. Rotate your shoulders forward, then back to the center, and backward for 30 seconds.

7 Stand in front of a wall or chair and use one hand for support. Keeping your right knee soft, bend your left leg, tucking your heel into your buttock. Clasp your foot with your left hand and hold for 10. Feel the stretch in your fron thigh. Change legs.

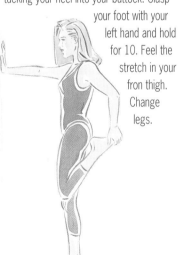

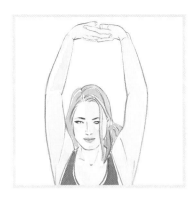

6 Stand and stretch your arms up so that they are either side of your ears. Link your fingertips and turn your palms toward the ceiling. Stretch and hold for a count of 8. Relax and repeat.

8 Stand with your legs wide apart, toes turned out. Make your hands into fists in front of your thighs. With stomach and buttocks tucked in, slowly bend your knees, keeping your heels on the floor, curling your arms up to your shoulders. Relax back into starting position and repeat for up to 1 minute.

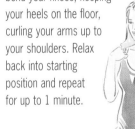

HELPFUL HEALTH TIPS

■ Frequency, not intensity, is the key to stretches. Ideally, try to do these warm-up exercises every morning when you wake up, even if you do not go on to do any other exercise.

■ To avoid post-exercise aches and pains, you must stretch out after you exercise, too, whether you have been doing stamina-building or toning exercises. See Cooling Down page 23.

■ Gentle daily exercise can help to prevent minor aches and pains and also help you to combat stress.

■ If you are very unfit, start your way to fitness by working up to three of these 10-minute warm-up sessions in a day. These short bursts of gentle exercise are easier to fit into your daily routine than one half-hour session. Studies have shown they may be better for promoting weight loss, too.

EffortlessExercise

Start getting fit by gently introducing exercise into your life. Here are some routines you can do around the house—waiting for a pot to boil or while watching a television program. All you need is a chair and tin cans or bottles of water to use as weights.

UPPER ARMS

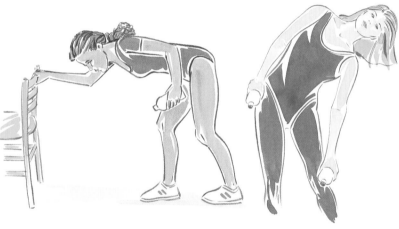

Stand an arm's length from a chair. Put your right foot in front of your left, hip-width apart. Keeping knees soft, lean forward from your hips until your body is parallel to the floor. Put your right hand on the chair for support. Holding a weight in your left hand, bend your left elbow and hold it close to your waist. Straighten your left arm behind you. Pause and bend back to starting position. Repeat 10 times, then change sides.

WAIST

Holding weights, stand upright, feet hip-width apart, arms resting down by your sides. Keep your back and shoulders straight and slowly bend at the waist down to the right without twisting. Try to reach your right hand down toward your ankle. Feel the stretch in your waist. Raise yourself up to the starting position, then stretch over to the left. Repeat the movement slowly up to 20 times on each side—do not bounce or jerk your body.

LEG STRETCHER

Do this simple exercise against the wall. Stretch your arms out in front of you at chest to shoulder level. Reach slowly forward as if someone is pulling your hands, but don't arch your back. Feel a slight stretch in the back of your legs and hold for 10 seconds. Return to the starting position and repeat the exercise up to 10 times.

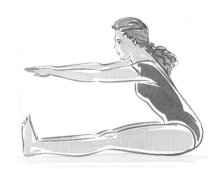

LEG SHAPER

Stand, feet hip-width apart, arms by your sides (use some weights to give you extra balance if you like). Lower your buttocks as if you are going to sit on a chair. Don't squat down too low and keep your heels on the floor. Slowly, slowly return to your starting position and repeat up to 10 times.

THIGH SHAPER

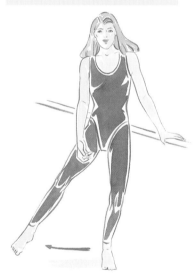

Hold the counter or the back of a chair with your left hand. Tighten your stomach and buttock muscles. Bend your left leg and lift your right foot out to the side. Keeping body tall, lift and lower the leg 10 times. Turn around and repeat.

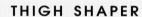

HELPFUL HEALTH TIPS

■ Turn the radio to a channel playing music with a beat, and dance or just jump around energetically for 2 minutes continuously. This will boost your heart rate, stamina, and circulation. It will also help to shake off stress and lethargy and warm you up for these simple stretching exercises.

■ Tone your legs while in the bathtub. Bend your left leg and stretch your right leg out in front. Raise and lower the right leg slowly 20 times. Swap legs.

■ Circle your wrists and ankles while lying in the bathtub. This is especially helpful to reduce swelling caused by fluid retention.

■ Wear loose, workout-style clothes when you're at home so you can settle down to some exercises whenever you have 10 minutes to spare. If you do nothing else, run briskly up and down stairs for 5 minutes at a time. This is excellent aerobic and firming exercise.

WorkWorkout

You can tone up flabby muscles, burn fat, and increase your energy levels on the way to work, sitting at your desk, and again on the way home. Try these toning exercises on the bus, train, or subway. If you work above the first floor, start taking the stairs instead of the elevator for a couple of flights and walk up them quickly. Your stamina and strength will soon increase if you do this twice daily for a couple of weeks—you'll soon be running up and down stairs!

UPPER BODY STRETCH

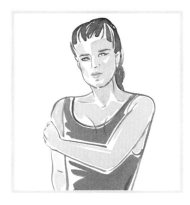 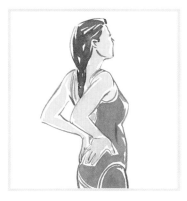

1 Sit upright in your chair, feet flat on the floor, your stomach muscles pulled in. Reach your left arm across the front of your body. Pull back your right arm to pull the left arm closer in to your chest. Feel the stretch in your left arm and shoulder. Hold for 10–15 seconds. Repeat with the right arm.

2 Stand up. Pull your stomach in tight and position your hands at the base of your back, just at the tops of buttocks. Slowly push your elbows closer together. Open up your chest to the ceiling and expand your rib cage. Hold for 10 seconds. Repeat 5 times. This exercise is good for relieving tension.

CHEST AND ARM FIRMER

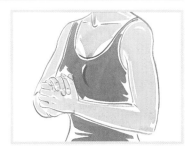

Sit with your hands, palms together, in your lap or in front of you at roughly waist height. Squeeze your palms together hard for a count of 5 and release. Repeat up to 10 times. This is a good exercise to do when you are stuck in a traffic jam.

THIGH TONER

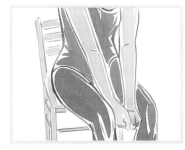

Tuck in your stomach muscles and sit tall. Make your hands into fists and place them between your knees. Alternatively, place a book bag or briefcase between your knees. Squeeze in with your thighs for a count of 50. Release and repeat.

BUTTOCK BUSTER

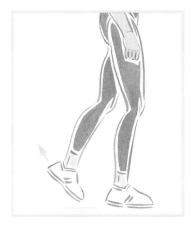

Do this exercise while you stand by the photocopier or coffee machine at work. Tighten your buttocks, hold in your stomach and, keeping your knees slightly bent and soft, move your left leg 2 in (5 cm) out behind you, with the foot off the floor. Hold for a count of 10, release and repeat on the other side. Alternate legs as long as you can.

HELPFUL HEALTH TIPS

■ Look slimmer and appear taller by improving your posture when walking or standing. You can do this anywhere. Stand up straight with your stomach and buttocks pulled in. If you hold this posture often enough, it will feel natural to you and you will feel odd when you slouch. The other benefits of improving your posture are improved muscle tone—your clothes will look better on you, too!

■ In your lunch break, take a brisk walk around town or swim for half an hour. This will improve your energy levels for the afternoon and will make you less likely to succumb to a mid-afternoon energy slump.

■ Walk briskly or bicycle all or part of the way to work— especially when the weather is good. You may find it an effort at first, but after a week or two you won't tire so easily.

UpperBodyTone

Exercise can seem like too much of an effort sometimes. Although you know that taking a walk would make you feel better, when it's cold or raining outside, it's hard to motivate yourself. If this sounds familiar, bring a little exercise into the bedroom. Experts say the best thing you can do to keep yourself in shape, and your metabolic rate boosted throughout the day, is to exercise frequently for short periods of time. Follow the warm-up routine on page 27 before beginning. Make sure your bed is firmly positioned so it won't slip during the exercises. You will also need a mat or towel to kneel on.

ARM SHAPERS

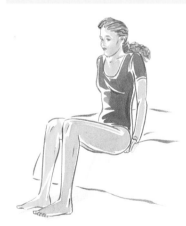 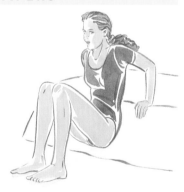

1 Sit on the edge of the bed, knees bent, toes pointing forward, and hands shoulder-width apart beneath your buttocks, gripping the bed for support.

2 Bend your arms as you lower your buttocks to the floor, holding your stomach in. Just before you reach the floor raise yourself back up, pushing down with your arms as you raise your body up. Repeat 10 times.

CHEST PRESS

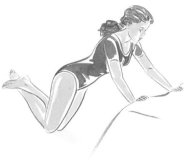 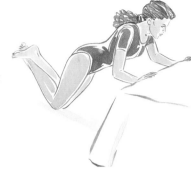

1 Kneel on the floor, on a folded towel if you need to. Position your hands on the bed slightly wider than shoulder-width apart, fingers pointing forward and then cross your ankles.

2 Lower your chest toward the bed. Keep your stomach pulled in and your body straight from head to knees. Push away from the bed. Repeat 10 times and work up to more.

WAIST CURLS

1 Lie on the floor with the lower part of your legs resting over the edge of the bed, your back pressed firmly into the floor. Loosely position your right hand behind your head and stretch your left hand out to the side.

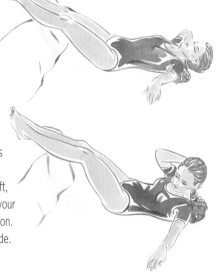

2 Pull in your abdominal muscles and curl up toward the bed, lifting from your waist. Twist to the left, leading with your right shoulder, not your elbow. Slowly return to starting position. Repeat 10 times. Repeat for other side.

TIPS

■ It is very important to breathe reasonably deeply and rhythmically when exercising. Be sure not to hold your breath while you concentrate on the exercise you are doing. If you find it difficult to breathe in and out as you exercise, count out loud each time you breathe out. If your breath gets short and breathing becomes an effort, it is time to slow down and not push yourself so hard. Don't worry, your stamina will improve rapidly if you exercise regularly.

■ Combine these exercises with Trimmer Arms on page 33, Chest Exercises on page 38, and Super Shoulders on page 40 for a complete upper body workout.

LowerBodyTone

Forget gyms and sweaty workout classes. You can work that body in the comfort of your own home until you are ready to go out and face the world. Begin by doing the energizing warm-up routine on page 27. You will need a couple of pillows and a mat or towel to lie on for this quick lower body workout.

SUPER SQUATS

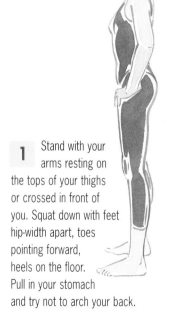 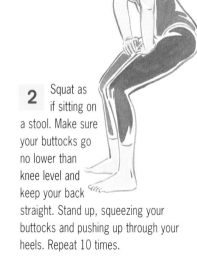

1 Stand with your arms resting on the tops of your thighs or crossed in front of you. Squat down with feet hip-width apart, toes pointing forward, heels on the floor. Pull in your stomach and try not to arch your back.

2 Squat as if sitting on a stool. Make sure your buttocks go no lower than knee level and keep your back straight. Stand up, squeezing your buttocks and pushing up through your heels. Repeat 10 times.

INNER THIGH SQUEEZE

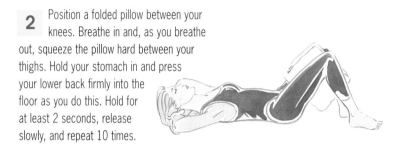

1 Lie on your back on the floor with your hands behind your head. Keep your knees bent and your feet slightly apart.

2 Position a folded pillow between your knees. Breathe in and, as you breathe out, squeeze the pillow hard between your thighs. Hold your stomach in and press your lower back firmly into the floor as you do this. Hold for at least 2 seconds, release slowly, and repeat 10 times.

STREAMLINED STOMACH

1 Lie on a mat on the floor with the lower part of your legs resting on the bed or sofa and your back pressed firmly into the floor. Loosely position your hands behind your head. (Never pull yourself up with your hands as this can strain your neck.)

2 Pull in your stomach, then slowly curl your body upward so that your head and shoulders, but not your lower back, leave the floor. Lower yourself back down. Repeat 10 times and build up to more.

HELPFUL HEALTH TIPS

■ Men and women store fat differently. Women tend to accumulate fat around their stomachs, hips, and thighs. This is why it is important to exercise these areas regularly. Exercise really helps to improve shape and muscle tone and to reduce the appearance of cellulite.

■ If you are totally new to exercise, you may find it hard to complete the recommended number of repetitions. Don't worry—increase the number of repetitions over a few sessions, working to the point where the muscle being trained feels slightly tired. Do one more repetition, then stop. Always listen to your body and stop if you feel tired or have any twinges or aches.

■ Combine these exercises with Better Buttocks on page 34, Inner Thigh Time on page 35, and Firm Outer Thighs on page 36 for a complete lower body workout.

Toned Stomach

Unlike leg and arm muscles, the abdominal, or stomach, muscles get little exercise in the course of a normal day. For this reason the stomach can quickly become slack and untoned. Women tend to store weight around the stomach, making the problem worse. The good news is that abdominal muscles respond well to exercise. With just a few targeted routines, you can quickly tone up your tummy. The key is to take your time—the slower you work, the more effective the results will be. Warm up by doing 3 minutes of marching in place, or, if you have time, begin by doing the warm-up routine on page 27. You will need a mat or towel to lie on.

STOMACH CURL

1 Lie on the floor with feet hip-width apart and your knees bent. Keep your back flat against the floor, tighten your stomach muscles, and gently raise your head and shoulders a few inches. Keep your chin off your chest throughout the exercise.

2 Slide your hands as far up toward your knees as you can, hold for a few seconds, then slowly return to starting position. Repeat 10 times, keeping the movement smooth, not jerky. As this exercise becomes easier, work up to 40 repetitions.

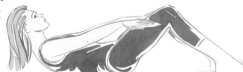

LOWER ABDOMEN CURL

1 Lie on the floor with your knees bent, feet hip-width apart. Put your arms, palms down, by your sides.

2 Raise your legs off the floor, and contract your stomach to lift your buttocks toward the ceiling, then lower them. Repeat 10 times and work up to 40. Keep your legs bent to make the exercise easier.

CRUNCH TIME

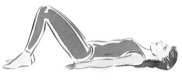

1 Lie on your back, knees bent and hip-width apart, feet on the floor. Tighten your stomach muscles and press your back firmly into the floor.

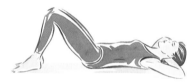

2 Place your hands loosely by the sides of your temples, with your elbows out to the sides. Keep your chin up—as if you have a small ball under it.

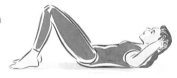

3 Keeping your neck straight and chin lifted, use your tightened stomach muscles to curl up, until your shoulder blades are off the floor.

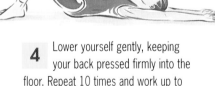

4 Lower yourself gently, keeping your back pressed firmly into the floor. Repeat 10 times and work up to 40 repetitions as this exercise becomes easier. Then stretch out your arms.

HELPFUL HEALTH TIPS

■ If you suffer from minor back aches and pains, weak abdominal muscles may be the cause. Do these stomach toning exercises three times a week to strengthen your stomach muscles. They will help improve poor posture, too. If you have back problems, always get professional advice before starting a new exercise program.

■ As you become more familiar with the exercises you can start controlling your breathing to make them more effective. For all these stomach exercises, breathe out as you lift your body and breathe in as you lower it.

■ It is important to hold your stomach muscles in as you do crunches—imagine your belly button is pressing down into your spine.

■ If your back does feel uncomfortable after exercise—or after a heavy shopping trip or just from sitting at a desk all day—try the Lower Back Soother on page 99.

Trimmer Arms

Trim, toned upper arms are not just for the young and super-fit. The exercises here strengthen the bicep and tricep (back of arm) muscles. You can tone up these muscles relatively quickly with a few simple, but regular, exercises. Do these three times a week or more and you should notice a difference in about one month. You will need a firm chair, a wall for support, and weights. March in place for a few minutes to warm up before you begin.

CHAIR DIP

1 Sit on the edge of a firm, stable chair. Keep your feet hip-width apart and hold onto the chair with your fingers gripping the edge of the seat.

2 Lower your buttocks slowly toward the floor, using your arms to support your weight. Ease back up, feeling the stretch in the back of your arms. Repeat 10 times, and build up to more.

WALL PUSH-UP

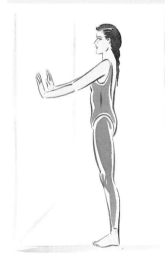 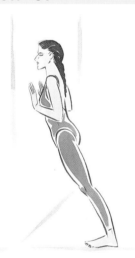

1 Stand facing a wall with your feet hip-width apart and your arms stretched out in front of you. Place your palms flat on the wall roughly in line with your rib cage.

2 Bend your elbows and push your body weight onto your arms, aiming your nose toward the wall and keeping your hips directly under your shoulders. Push out. Repeat 10 times.

BICEP CURLS

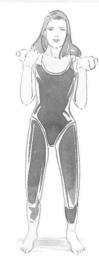 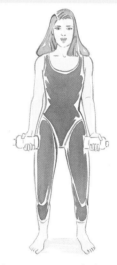

1 Stand with feet hip-width apart, knees soft. With a weight in each hand, bend your arms at the elbows, then bring them up to your shoulders, keeping your elbows close to your body.

2 Lower your arms slowly to the starting position, making sure your elbows do not lock as you lower and extend your arms. Repeat the exercise 10 times.

HELPFUL HEALTH TIPS

■ Combine bicep curls with squats for an upper and lower body workout. Squat down as though you are going to sit on a low stool (for an illustration of this see Super Squats on page 31). As you do so, bend your elbows and bring your forearms into your chest. Return to the starting position and repeat 10 times, building up to more repetitions.

■ Breathe out on the hardest part of each exercise. Breathe in as you go down in dips and curls and as you bend your elbows during push-ups; breathe out with the effort of returning to the starting position.

■ The skin around the tops of your arms can get dimply due to cellulite or it may be bumpy and dull due to poor skin tone and lack of exfoliation. For ways to improve the condition of your skin, check out Section 5— Look Good.

BetterButtocks

To get your buttocks into shape, try these simple but powerful exercises. Do the warm-up routine on page 27 or march in place for a few minutes before you begin. For the leg lunges and buttock toner, work on a non-slip surface.

BUTTOCK BEATER

1 Put a towel or mat on the floor and position yourself on your knees, resting the upper part of your body on your elbows. Holding your stomach muscles in tightly, bend one leg up, flexing the foot. Keeping the foot flexed, lift the knee upward toward the ceiling until you feel the buttocks contract. Lower the leg and repeat 10 times. Next, hold the raised leg position and "pulse" the leg upward, making small, fast movements for a count of 10.

2 Now squeeze up and move the heel inward, approximately 6 in (15 cm), toward your buttocks. First lift the leg, curl in the heel, then release and lower slightly. Repeat 10 times. Do the entire sequence on the other leg.

LEG LUNGES

1 Stand with feet hip-width apart. Turn your left foot in slightly. Step forward about 3 feet (90 cm) with your right foot. Check your hips are facing forward. Relax your shoulders, lift your chest, and contract your stomach and buttocks.

2 Breathe in and lower your left thigh and bend your right knee. Make sure your right knee does not go in front of your toes and your rear end does not drop below the line of your knee. Return to the starting position and repeat 10 times, working alternate legs.

BUTTOCK TONER

1 Stand behind a firm chair or work surface with feet hip-width apart. Pull in your stomach and buttocks. Go onto tiptoes, hold for a few seconds, and lower. Repeat 10 times.

2 Stand with feet shoulder-width apart and toes out. Go on tiptoes and bend your knees, keeping your back straight and taking your buttocks no lower than the knees. Lower heels to the floor. Repeat 10 times.

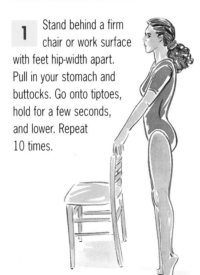

■ Take the stairs whenever you can and take them two at a time. This will give your buttocks an effective mini-workout.

■ Whenever you find yourself standing during the day (standing in line, or on the bus, or while ironing, for example), clench your buttocks tightly and release. Aim to do this as often as you can, and there should be a noticeable improvement in muscle tone within weeks.

■ Lunges are excellent for toning buttocks, but it is essential that you don't put any stress on the knees and back. Do not step so far forward or backward that you cannot return to standing without putting pressure on the lower back or losing your balance or posture. Do the exercises in front of a mirror occasionally so you can check your posture.

Inner ThighTime

Inner thighs are prone to flabbiness, and most women would like to firm them up. These exercises will tighten and tone up the area and improve circulation. Warm up before starting by marching in place for a few minutes or doing the warm-up sequence on page 27. You will need a mat or towel to lie on, and a firm chair for support.

INNER THIGH RAISE

1 Lie on your right side, propped up on your right forearm. Breathe regularly.

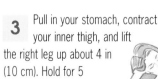

2 Bend your left knee, placing your foot flat on the floor in front of the right leg. Flex your right foot and extend the leg so the inner thigh faces the ceiling.

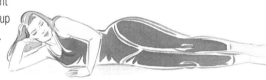

3 Pull in your stomach, contract your inner thigh, and lift the right leg up about 4 in (10 cm). Hold for 5 seconds and lower. Repeat 10 times. Change legs.

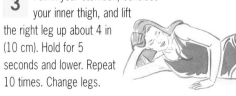

INNER THIGH PRESS

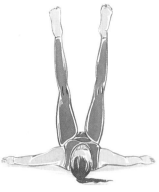
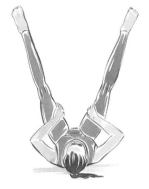

1 Lie on your back. Raise your legs slowly, keeping your knees slightly bent. Make sure your neck is relaxed and your head on the floor.

2 Place your hands on the insides of your thighs. Hold in your abdominals, pushing out with your hands while you push in with your thighs.

BASIC PLIÉ

1 Hold on to the back of a chair. Stand up straight with your feet a little wider than shoulder-width apart and your feet turned out slightly.

2 Keeping your heels on the floor and your buttocks tucked in, slowly bend your knees, making sure your buttocks go no lower than your knees. Repeat up to 10 times.

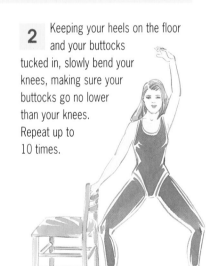

■ Cellulite particularly affects the inner thigh area. To combat it, check out the information in War On Cellulite on page 119.

■ Pliés are excellent leg and buttock toners. To make them even more effective, squeeze your inner thighs and buttock muscles as you raise yourself up. There are more ballet-style exercises on page 45.

■ You can work your inner thighs while sitting in front of the television. Put a pillow between your knees, squeeze hard, and release. Repeat as many times as you can.

FirmOuterThighs

The outer thighs are a major problem area for many women. Make yours look leaner and more shapely by doing the warm-up routine on page 27, then tackling these three simple exercises. Stand on a non-slip surface for the outer thigh lift. Use a mat or towel to lie on for the other exercises.

OUTER THIGH LIFT

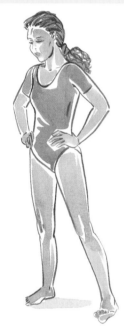 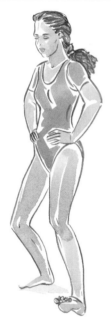

1 Stand with feet shoulder-width apart and hands on a chair or your hip bones. Lift left leg out to the side keeping your foot flexed. Hold for a count of 5. Return to starting position.

2 Slowly bend your knees, as though you are going to sit down on a low stool. Raise your left leg and hold for a count of 5. Repeat the exercise 10 times on each leg.

OUTER THIGH RAISE

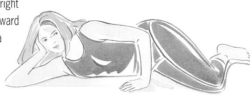

1 Lie on your right side, propped up on your right forearm, leaning slightly forward and with your legs bent at a 45-degree angle.

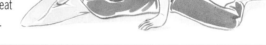

2 Raise your left leg, keeping it parallel to the ceiling, using the outer thigh muscle to do the work. Return to starting position. Repeat 10 times on each leg.

OUTER THIGH STRETCH

1 Lie on your back with your knees bent, feet flat on the floor, and your hands palms down by your sides. Lift your left leg and rest your ankle on your right thigh, just above the knee.

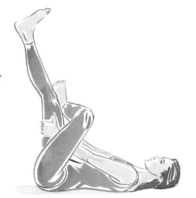

2 For a bigger stretch, lift your right leg as high as you can, supporting your right thigh with both hands. Keep your head as close to the floor as possible. Pull your right leg in gently until you feel the stretch. Use your right leg to push the left leg forward to stretch the outer thigh and gluteal (buttock) muscles. Hold for a count of 5. Repeat 10 times on both legs.

HELPFUL HEALTH TIPS

■ To see quick results, do these exercises once or twice daily.

■ Do toning exercises at a variety of tempos—ultraslow and then pulsing more quickly—to get the maximum benefit from the movements.

■ Build up the number of repetitions slowly. You might not be able to do the whole routine at the first attempt. After doing the routine regularly for a few weeks, you'll find that you are up to the suggested number of repetitions. Then you can add more, making sure you are listening to your body all the time to be certain you aren't putting it under any strain.

■ Firm up your whole lower body by following up these exercises with those explained in Inner Thigh Time on page 35 and Better Buttocks on page 34.

■ Aerobic exercise, such as dancing, will help keep your lower body in trim, too. See Section 1—Get Moving!

LeanerLegs

Legs get a workout if you walk occasionally instead of taking the car. There are, however, useful targeted exercises you can do to make your legs shapelier. March in place for a few minutes to warm up before starting. You will need a wall for support, a mat or towel to lie on, and, if you want to add to the effectiveness of the moves, tin cans or bottles of water to use as weights.

FRONT OF LEG SHAPER

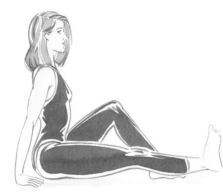

1 Sit on the floor with your left leg bent, the right leg flat on the floor. Place your hands behind your buttocks with palms flat on the floor. Lean against a wall if you need extra support for your back.

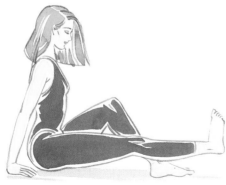

2 Hold in your abdominal muscles and extend the right leg, with foot flexed and toes pointing toward the ceiling. Then slowly raise it about 2–3 in (5–7 cm) off the floor and lower it. Repeat 10 times and change legs.

BEND AND STRAIGHTEN

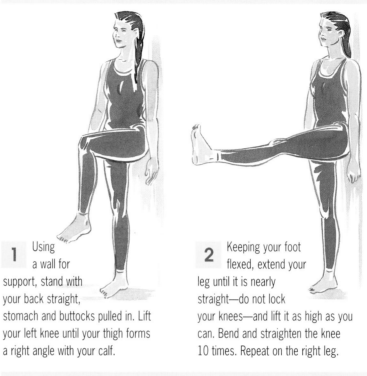

1 Using a wall for support, stand with your back straight, stomach and buttocks pulled in. Lift your left knee until your thigh forms a right angle with your calf.

2 Keeping your foot flexed, extend your leg until it is nearly straight—do not lock your knees—and lift it as high as you can. Bend and straighten the knee 10 times. Repeat on the right leg.

THIGH PRESS AND LIFT

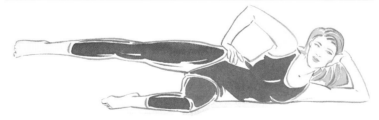

Lie on your side with your head supported on your hand, elbow on the floor. Pull your abdominals in. Bend your lower leg slightly and keep the top leg straight and in line with your hip and shoulder. Flex your foot and point your toes down. Use your outer thigh muscle to lift your top leg about 1 in (2.5 cm) above the line of your hip. Lower to the floor. Repeat 10 times, then change sides.

HELPFUL HEALTH TIPS

■ To give calves and ankles a workout, try to walk around barefoot as much as you can. Walking barefoot on sand is especially beneficial.

■ If you suffer from puffy ankles in the heat or because you have to stand a lot, rotate your ankles several times in both directions to reduce the swelling. This helps to reduce puffiness when you're traveling by airplane, too.

■ Walking is great exercise for the legs and puts less strain on the body than jogging. Check out the information in Walk Yourself Fit on page 18 and Power Walking on page 19.

■ The shins of the legs contain no sebaceous, or oil-producing, glands, which is why you tend to have dry, flaky skin around this area. To help improve the look and feel of your legs, see Body Care on page 118.

Chest**Exercises**

All women want a firm, toned bust. Exercise cannot make the bust bigger because there is no muscle in the breasts, but you can firm up the surrounding area and give your breasts extra support. Warm up by marching in place for a couple of minutes. You will need a mat or towel to lie on, and weights.

PALM CLASPS

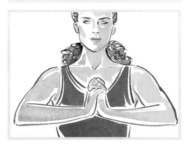

Stand with your feet hip-width apart and the palms of your hands together in front of your chest, fingers interlinked. Pull in and tighten your abdominal muscles. Press your palms together hard and hold for 5 seconds. Repeat the exercise up to 10 times.

ELBOW PRESSES

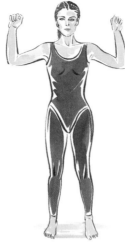

1 Stand with your feet hip-width apart, knees slightly bent, arms raised out to your sides. Keep elbows bent and hands in soft "fists."

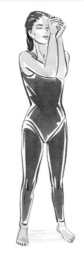

2 Slowly bring your elbows and forearms in so they are pressing together in front of your chest. Repeat the exercise up to 10 times.

ELBOW CROSSES

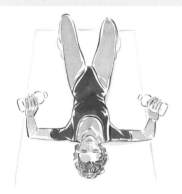

1 Lie flat on your back, knees bent, feet flat on the floor, holding the weights with your elbows bent.

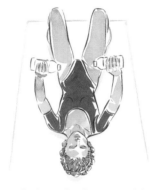

2 Push your hands up toward the ceiling. Your palms should be facing forward, toward your thighs.

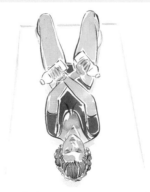

3 Slowly move your arms toward each other, so that your elbows cross above your chest.

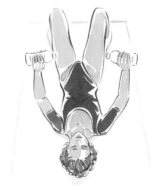

4 Slowly lower your arms. Repeat up to 10 times, alternating the arm crossing over at the top.

TIPS

■ Try to avoid rapid weight loss or gain as this can stretch the delicate breast tissue leading to sagging.

■ The skin from the chin to the base of the breasts is thin, mainly due to the weight of the bust. This area is therefore prone to wrinkles, and you should protect and look after it as you would the skin on your face. Always use plenty of protective sunscreen when out in the sun and moisturize regularly. For more healthy skin tips see Section 5—Look Good.

■ A simple trick to keep breasts pert and help prevent them from drooping is to spray them daily with cold water while taking a shower.

■ The chest can be prone to pimples because of the high number of sebaceous glands in that area. Include the chest in your usual cleansing routine and see Pimple Attack on page 108.

Waist**Workshop**

Weight and extra inches go onto the waist all too easily as we get older. Fortunately, it's also easy to trim your waist with a combination of a low-fat diet and a simple sequence of exercises. You will need a mat or towel to lie on, and tin cans or bottles of water to use as weights.

TWIST AND STRETCH

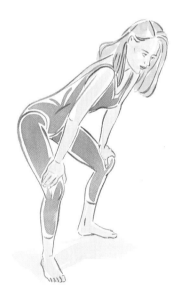

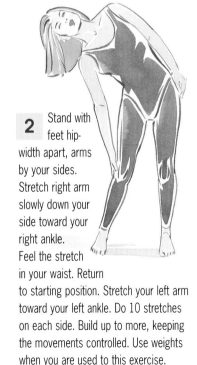

1 First warm up the lower back (see page 27). Bend forward about 30 degrees, placing your hands above your kneecaps to support your back. Round out gently and then straighten your spine 8 times.

2 Stand with feet hip-width apart, arms by your sides. Stretch right arm slowly down your side toward your right ankle. Feel the stretch in your waist. Return to starting position. Stretch your left arm toward your left ankle. Do 10 stretches on each side. Build up to more, keeping the movements controlled. Use weights when you are used to this exercise.

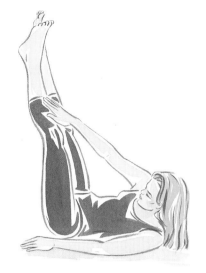

3 Lie on your back, pressing your lower back firmly into the floor and tightening your stomach muscles. Raise your legs straight up in front of you, keeping the knees slightly bent. Stretch toward your left foot with your right hand, then toward your right foot with your left hand. Use your abdominals, not your neck or back, to do the work. Reach up to alternate sides 20 times (10 on each side.) Rest for 5 seconds and try another set of 20 "reaches."

4 Lie on your back with your knees bent. Put your right foot on your left knee. Place your left hand under your head at the nape of your neck. Hold in your abdominals, lift up and twist to the right, leading with your shoulder not your elbow. Return to the starting position. Repeat on the other side. Do 10 repetitions on each side.

5 Lie on your back with your knees bent, feet on the floor, your arms down by your sides and your fingertips pointing toward your toes. Contract your abdominals and raise your head and shoulders slightly off the floor. Continue to contract your stomach muscles and push your right hand toward your right foot. Repeat on the other side. Alternate up to 10 times.

HELPFUL HEALTH **TIPS**

■ Choose clothes carefully to highlight your good physical features and disguise problem areas. If you don't have a well-defined waist, for example, looser, low-slung trousers are more flattering. Avoid pleated pants and go for flat-fronted styles. Fitted shirts and jackets that are nipped in at the waist help give the illusion of a slim waist. But don't try pulling yourself in with wide belts—they emphasize a lack of waist.

■ Improving the muscle tone of your shoulders and upper body will help define your waist. Try doing the Super Shoulders routine on page 40. Add a weekly swim to your fitness and exercise routine to supplement this upper body workout.

Super**Shoulders**

Exercising your shoulders can improve the shape of your body, making your shoulders look slightly wider, your waist look smaller, and giving your upper body more of a "triangular" shape. Most of us don't worry about our shoulders because it is not an area that accumulates fat, but it is worth trying these routines to improve your shape and flexibility. March in place for a few minutes to warm up. You will need a mat or towel to lie on. Use water bottles or tin cans for weights to increase the effectiveness of the exercises.

SHOULDER PRESSES

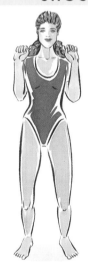 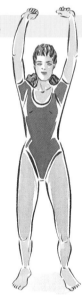

1 Stand with feet hip-width apart, knees soft, arms down to the sides, elbows bent, and hands at shoulder height. Hold in abdominals and buttocks.

2 Slowly push your arms up straight with your palms toward the ceiling. Do not lock your elbows. Slowly lower your arms. Repeat 10 times.

PULL-UPS

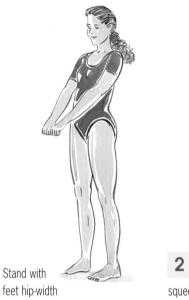

1 Stand with feet hip-width apart, arms forward, elbows at waist height. Hold in abdominals and buttocks.

2 Pull your elbows back and squeeze between the shoulder blades as you pull arms up to shoulder level. Return to starting position. Repeat 10 times.

PUSH-UPS

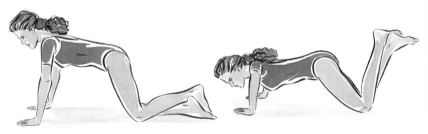

1 On a mat or towel on the floor, position yourself on your knees, feet on the floor and ankles crossed. Place your arms directly under your shoulders, hands straight out in front.

2 Using your arms, lower yourself slowly toward the floor as far as you can, pulling in your stomach and buttock muscles. Repeat 10 times. As you get stronger, keep your feet off the floor.

HELPFUL HEALTH TIPS

■ Most of us carry one shoulder higher than the other, as a result of tensing the area through stress, and doing things such as holding the telephone receiver between jaw and shoulder, and carrying a heavy bag on one side. Learn to relax your shoulders, avoid cradling the telephone receiver against your shoulder, and when carrying things try to distribute the weight evenly.

■ To relieve tension in the shoulders, try the Desk Stretchers on page 84. These simple stretches can be done at your desk or on a long journey.

■ The skin on the shoulders and the back often gets neglected and may be dull-looking or suffer from spots. Exfoliate regularly to keep skin looking good. Check out Body Care on page 118.

PearShaped?

Your genes largely determine how much you can change your body shape. They also dictate where you tend to carry fat and muscle. The two most common body shapes are "apples" and "pears." Apples carry excess weight around the middle. Pears carry weight around the hips and thighs. Dieting can accentuate a pear shape rather than improving it because the top half shrinks as much as the bottom half, leaving a smaller pear! So pears need to focus on lower body toning exercises like these. You will need a mat or towel to kneel and lie on for this toning routine. Start with the short warm-up on page 27 to get your body moving.

BUTTOCK CLENCHER

1 Lie on your stomach and put a folded towel under your hips to prevent your back from curving. Rest your head on your arms.

2 Clench your buttocks and curl one leg in, with foot flexed. Lift your knee 2 in (5 cm) off the floor. Hold for a count of one and lower. Do 10 lifts on each leg.

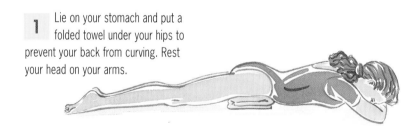

INNER THIGH TIGHTENER

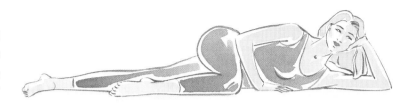

1 Lie on your left side, back straight, and tummy held in. Keep your left leg straight, bend your right knee, and rest it on the floor in front of you.

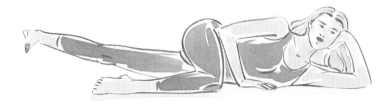

2 Breathe out and lift your left (underneath) leg as high as you can, keeping your foot flexed and your stomach held in. Repeat 10 times on each side.

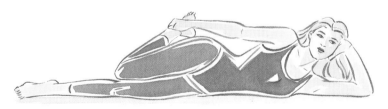

3 To stretch out the thighs, relax your left leg so it's flat on the floor. Use your right hand to pull the right ankle toward your buttocks. Keep the knees together and push the right hip forward. Hold for 20 seconds. Repeat on the other side.

HELPFUL HEALTH TIPS

■ To help keep weight off the hip and thigh area, you need to do aerobic exercise. Check out the routines in Section 1—Get Moving! If you enjoy walking or bicycling, these activities will also help slim your hips and thighs.

■ Most women are pears and tend to store fat around the hip and thigh area. Keeping your diet low in fat will help you to avoid storing more fat in these areas. The Fat Facts on page 54 will give you some useful tips.

■ For more exercises to firm up hips and thighs, see Inner Thigh Time on page 35 and Firm Outer Thighs on page 36.

■ If you are more apple-shaped than pear-shaped, concentrate your exercise time on toning up your stomach muscles—see Toned Stomach on page 32.

FacialWorkout

Your face can benefit from exercise too. Toning your facial muscles can help prevent sagging, improve circulation and skin tone, and reduce double chins and puffy, baggy eyes. Do these simple exercises for a few minutes twice a day and you will see positive results in just a few weeks.

A DEFINED CHIN

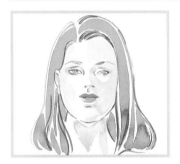

1 Sit up straight with your chin held high. Close your lips tightly together and try to smile using only your upper lip.

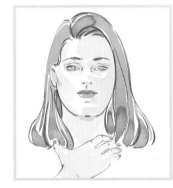

2 Place one hand at the base of your throat over the collar bone and pull down slightly on the skin with a firm grip.

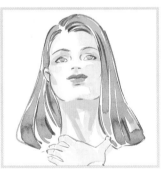

3 Tilt your head back gently and you will feel a strong pull on the chin and neck muscles. Return your head to the starting position and repeat steps 2 and 3 around 30 times.

EYE OPENERS

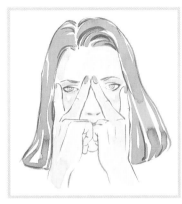
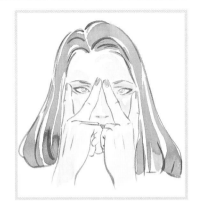

1 Place your middle fingers between your eyebrows, just above the bridge of the nose. Position your index fingers at the outer corners of your eyes.

2 Roll your eyes up and look at an imaginary line down the center of your forehead. Repeat and release 10 times. Keep looking up and in and squeeze your eyelids shut for a count of 40.

SCULPTURED CHEEKS

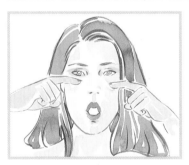
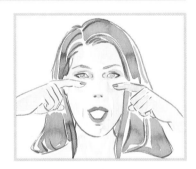

1 Position your index fingers on top of each cheekbone. Open your mouth, pushing the top and bottom lips apart to form a long "O" shape.

2 Hold the "O" shape, keeping your upper lip pressed against your top teeth. Smile with the corners of your mouth and release. Repeat 5 times, feeling the cheek muscles move.

HELPFUL HEALTH TIPS

■ Make these exercises part of your daily skin-cleansing routine—you'll be able to see what you're doing in the mirror. Alternatively, when you have mastered the techniques and can do the exercises without a mirror, you can do the routine while relaxing in the bath.

■ Another quick exercise to work your face is to raise your eyebrows as high as they will go, keeping the rest of your face still. Hold for a count of 5, lower, and repeat for about 1 minute.

■ Feeding your skin with the right nutrients will improve its condition. See the juicing ideas on pages 58 and 59. "Water" your skin by drinking 6 to 8 glasses of water a day, too.

■ Pamper your face with some quick-and-easy beauty treatments. Turn to Section 5—Look Good for the Fantastic Fast Facial on page 111 and Ten-minute Masks on page 112.

Age-defying Plan

As early as your late twenties, the telltale signs of aging will start to show. After the age of 30, the body begins to lose bone mass and muscles lose tone. Many of us take less exercise and are therefore more prone to gain weight that seems difficult to lose. But don't despair! Whatever your age, you can get stronger, leaner, and look younger with this simple tone-up routine. It targets the key problem areas—stomach, upper arms, buttocks, and hips. Take a brisk 5-minute walk to warm up before exercising or follow the warm-up routine on page 27. You will need a mat or towel to lie and kneel on.

TOTAL STOMACH TONER

1 Lie on your back with your knees bent, heels raised near the backs of your thighs. Place your hands behind your head, neck relaxed, and elbows comfortably out to the side. Breathe out and tighten your abdominals.

2 Raise legs in the air with knees slightly bent. Simultaneously, pull your rib cage toward your hips by lifting your head, neck, and shoulders and pull in your stomach muscles so your buttocks lift off the floor slightly. Hold for a few seconds. Lower your body, then your legs. Repeat the exercise 10 times.

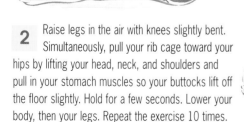

UPPER ARM SHAPER

1 Position yourself on your hands and knees with your body straight and your wrists lined up under your shoulders, fingers turned in slightly.

2 Breathe in and bend your elbows, lowering your body until your chest nears the floor. Keep your stomach pulled in tight. Pause, breathe out, and push back up to starting position. Repeat 10 times.

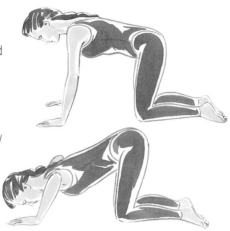

BUTTOCKS AND HIPS

1 Stand up straight with your stomach muscles tightened, feet hip-width apart, and hands at your sides. Check that your shoulders and neck are relaxed.

2 Breathe in, bend your knees as if you are going to sit in a chair, and slowly lower yourself until your thighs are nearly parallel to the floor. Hold your arms in front of you. Hold for a few seconds, breathe out, and slowly stand up. Repeat 10 times.

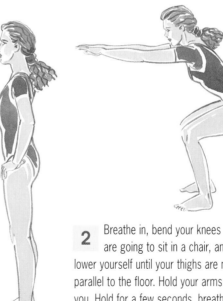

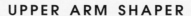

HELPFUL HEALTH TIPS

■ The Total Stomach Toner is a tough exercise. You may need to build up your abdominal muscles more gradually by starting with the simple crunches and curls shown on page 32.

■ When the age-defying exercises become easy, repeat the complete sequence twice and build up to three times.

■ As you get older, your body's ability to absorb calcium is decreased. To help maintain healthy bones, eat a diet with plenty of calcium-rich foods. These include low-fat dairy products, leafy green vegetables, beans, nuts, and canned fish with softened bones, such as canned salmon or sardines. Exercise regularly to improve bone density, and get plenty of daylight, which helps your body produce vitamin D.

■ Regular exercise, dealing effectively with stress, eating well, cutting down on alcohol, not smoking, and looking after your skin will all help you look younger.

Minimal Moves

Some fitness experts and dance and movement teachers believe that the best, and most effective, type of exercise is small, controlled movements that tone the muscles deep down. To those watching, it might seem that you are barely moving. The good thing about this type of exercise is that it forces you to concentrate on the muscle being worked. Bear in mind that you need to make a lot of tiny controlled movements for maximum results. You will need a mat or towel to lie on and a firm chair for support during this routine.

HIPS, BUTTOCKS, & THIGH TIGHTENER

1 Stand with feet together, hands resting on the back of a chair. Take your right leg out to the side, flexing your foot and pointing your toes toward the floor. Bend your left knee slightly.

2 Move your hips to the left slightly, bring your right leg in and tighten your buttocks. Move your right leg up and down just ¼ in (5 mm). Repeat 25 times, then work the other side.

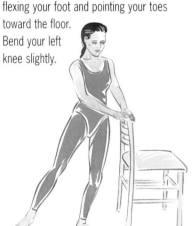
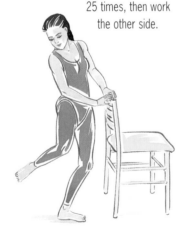

ARM TONER

1 Stand erect, feet hip-width apart. Bend your knees slightly. Take your arms up and out to the side, keeping them straight and in line with your shoulders. Slowly rotate your hands backward so your palms and thumbs face the ceiling. Tighten your buttocks and abdomen.

2 Curl your pelvis up. Move your arms behind your back, keeping your hands roughly level with your shoulders and your arms straight. With tiny movements move your arms ¼ in (5 mm) upwards. Repeat at least 25 times, and build up to 50.

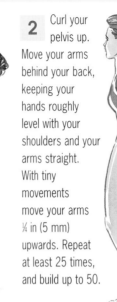
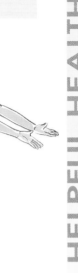

STOMACH TIGHTENER

1 Lie on the floor, knees bent, feet hip-width apart, arms by your sides. Gradually curl up, using your stomach muscles to lift you and raise your head and shoulders off the floor.

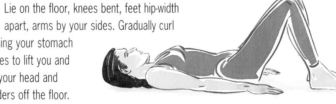

2 Keeping stomach tight and head raised, lift your arms 6 in (15 cm) off the floor. In slow motion move your hands ¼ in (5 mm) toward your feet and then back again. Repeat this tiny movement 25 times and aim for 50 repetitions.

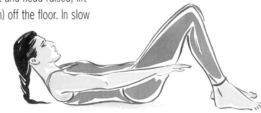

HELPFUL HEALTH TIPS

■ The slow, controlled movements described here require concentration. Think very carefully about the muscle you are working as you do each exercise to help make the movements as effective as possible. Try to keep your breathing smooth and even.

■ Slow exercises that isolate particular muscle groups can help you to build muscle strength relatively quickly if you practice the movements at least three times a week.

■ Having good posture—head held high, body erect, yet relaxed—can help you to look stronger, leaner, and firmer. The exercises on this page will help you become more conscious of your muscle strength and to improve your posture. See also Posture Improvers on page 47.

Ballet Style

Dancers' bodies always look lean, strong, and incredibly graceful. Dancers also move with great poise and have excellent posture. Try these simple movements based on ballet exercises to make your body stronger and more flexible and help improve your posture.

BALLETIC STRETCH

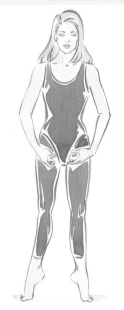 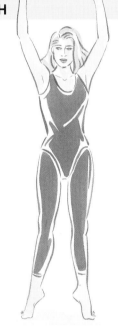

1 Stand with your heels together, toes pointing out, arms in front of you held loosely at hip level. Breathe in deeply, then breathe out as you tighten your abdominals and buttocks, and rise onto the balls of your feet.

2 Extend your arms gracefully overhead, keeping your shoulders down and relaxed. Breathe in as you slowly release your feet back down to the floor. Repeat the exercise up to 10 times.

DEMI-PLIÉ

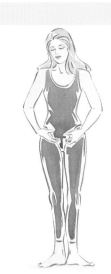 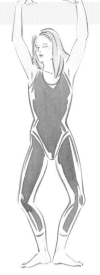

1 Stand with heels together, toes pointing out, arms held loosely in front of you. Breathe in and bend your knees, keeping your feet flat on the floor.

2 Extend your arms gracefully overhead. Breathe out and squeeze your buttocks and thighs as you return to standing. Repeat 10 times.

EXTENDED PLIÉ

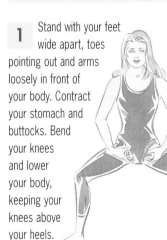

1 Stand with your feet wide apart, toes pointing out and arms loosely in front of your body. Contract your stomach and buttocks. Bend your knees and lower your body, keeping your knees above your heels.

2 Place your left hand on your left thigh and lean to the left. Extend your right arm over your head. Hold for 20 seconds. Repeat 5 times on each side.

HELPFUL HEALTH TIPS

■ In all these ballet-style exercises, make sure your weight is evenly distributed through your feet and that you are able to wiggle your toes, indicating that your feet are relaxed.

■ Do these exercises in front of a mirror so you can check your posture and the alignment of your body.

■ If you find it hard to balance on tiptoe, concentrate on looking at a fixed, still point in front of you.

■ T'ai Chi is an exercise program that employs a similar graceful and tranquil style. If you enjoy ballet-style exercises, you might also enjoy this eastern form of exercise. Check out classes in your area.

■ Stretching exercises, such as Stretch Slimmer on page 46 and Stress-Relieving Stretches on page 96, combine well with these ballet exercises if you want to extend the routine.

StretchSlimmer

To help you lengthen shortened muscles and loosen tight ones, try these simple stretches. They are ideal if your body has become rather inflexible through lack of exercise. So if touching your toes has become a distant memory—get stretching! You will notice an improvement surprisingly quickly. The other good news is that you will develop a longer, leaner, trimmer body.

SIDE STRETCHES

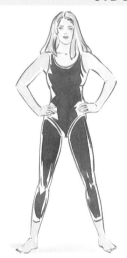 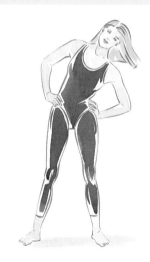

1 Stand with your feet shoulder-width apart, your knees soft and slightly bent. Keep your hands on your waist and your hips and legs still throughout the exercise for maximum effect. Breathe steadily.

2 Bend your upper body to the left slowly and gently. Keep the movement controlled. Return to upright, then bend to the right, feeling the stretch in your waist. Return to upright. Repeat the movement up to 10 times.

SHOULDER STRETCH

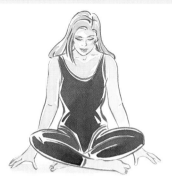 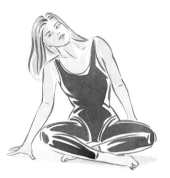

1 Sit on the floor with your legs crossed comfortably in front of you. Spread your fingers on the floor by your sides for support. Breathe regularly.

2 Look ahead and tilt head to the right. Feel the stretch in your neck. Rotate your left shoulder clockwise and counter-clockwise. Repeat on other side.

LOWER BODY STRETCH

1 Lie on your front and turn your head sideways, relax your shoulders, and point your right arm forward. Bend your left knee and hold at the ankle with your left hand. Ease your leg into the buttock. Feel the stretch in the hip and thigh. Hold for 20 seconds and change legs.

2 Lie on your back and make a diamond shape with your legs—soles of feet together and knees dropping out to sides. Hold for 20 seconds. Apply a little pressure with your hands to your inner thighs to increase the stretch. Relax and repeat.

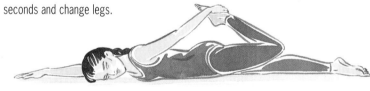

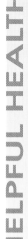

■ Combining a stretching routine with aerobic activity will increase the effectiveness of both activities. You will find you can stretch much farther after you have exercised and your muscles are warm. Stretching also prevents muscular aches and pains after you've worked your muscles hard aerobically.

■ Aches and pains when you wake up are not simply a natural sign of aging. They are also due to tension collecting in the muscles. Mental stress, as well as unusual physical exertion, makes muscles tense. You may not notice the tension during the day while you are moving around, but it can accumulate during sleep. The key to avoiding morning aches is to stretch out before you go to bed. This relaxes your mind and your body. Check out the Stress-relieving Stretches on page 96 and the Essential Daily Relaxation routine on page 98. You can also stretch out very gently in bed before you get up.

PostureImprovers

Improving your posture can have excellent effects. You will look and feel taller, more confident, and slimmer—instantly. Good posture is also the first step to having a pain-free back. It's never too late to get into good habits, stop slumping, and do what your teachers told you—sit up straight! The key to proper spine support is to position your pelvis in a central position. Your knees should be relaxed, and there should be a slight natural curve to your lower back. These exercises will help adjust your pelvis to its correct position. You will need a firm, straight-backed chair.

THE PELVIC TILT

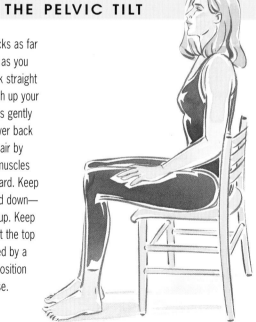

Sit with your buttocks as far back into the chair as you can. Try to keep your back straight and do not slouch or hunch up your shoulders. Rest your hands gently on your lap. Push your lower back against the back of the chair by tightening the abdominal muscles and tilting your pelvis upward. Keep your shoulders relaxed and down—not hunched up or raised up. Keep your chin up—imagine that the top of your head is being pulled by a piece of string. Hold the position for 10 seconds and release. Repeat several times.

POSTURE CORRECTOR

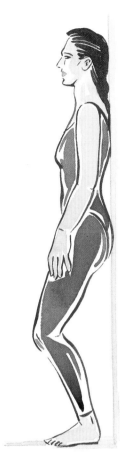
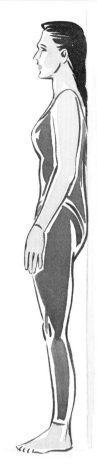

1 Lean against a wall, knees bent, feet hip-width apart and heels 6 in (15 cm) from the wall. Let your shoulders and buttocks touch the wall. Close the gap between the small of your back and the wall by pressing the base of the spine into the wall and pulling in your stomach.

2 Slowly straighten your legs and push your back up the wall, keeping your chin level and the back of your head against the wall. Hold for a count of 10. Repeat the routine 3 times. Aim to follow this posture correction routine every day for 2 weeks.

HELPFUL HEALTH TIPS

■ Use a footrest when sitting at a desk—a telephone directory or thick book will do the trick.

■ Sit as far back in a chair as you can to keep your back straight and supported. Get up and move around every half hour. When standing up from a seated position, straighten your back first and lead with your head.

■ Pack heavy shopping in two bags rather than one, hold one in each hand, and bend your knees, not your back, to lift them. If you only have one bag of groceries, hold it in front of you above hip level. Avoid holding heavy boxes or bags low in front of your pelvis.

■ Strong abdominals are essential for good posture. For exercises to strengthen the abdominal muscles, see Toned Stomach on page 32. Swimming strengthens the abs and back, too. Check out Water Workout on page 22 for simple exercises you can do in the pool.

BackBasics

Joints rely on movement for lubrication, and ligaments and muscles tighten and tense if they are not stretched. Exercising and stretching your back regularly will help prevent everyday aches and pains. You will need a mat or towel to lie on, and tin cans or bottles of water to use as weights.

SHOULDERS AND UPPER BACK

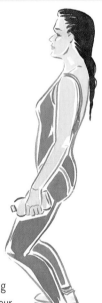

1 Stand with knees relaxed, palms facing your thighs. Bring your shoulders back and squeeze the shoulder blades and upper back muscles as you move your hands around and up from your thighs to the sides of your hips.

2 Shrug the shoulders as close to your ears as you can. Release and bring your hands back to your thighs. Repeat at least 10 times. Use weights to increase the effectiveness of the exercise.

STRETCH OUT

1 Lie on your back with your arms outstretched at shoulder level. Tighten your abdominal muscles. Raise your left leg slowly.

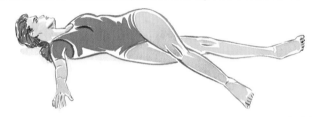

2 Move your left leg across the right leg. Keep shoulders and back pressed into the floor. Hold for 5 seconds. Repeat with other leg. Do the sequence 5 times.

A STRONGER SPINE

1 Lie face down, arms by your sides and close to body, forehead touching the floor. Raise your head and shoulders. Hold for 5 seconds. Repeat, with hands behind your head. Hold for 5 seconds and relax. Do not raise your head and shoulders any higher than is comfortable.

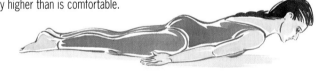

2 Raise your head and shoulders and each leg in turn, hold for 5 seconds, and relax.

HELPFUL HEALTH TIPS

■ Swimming may help relieve back pain because it strengthens the abdominals and supports the spine. However, doing the breast stroke while keeping your head above water makes you arch your lower back and could aggravate lower back and neck problems. If you enjoy swimming but are not sure about your swimming style, take some lessons.

■ Do not bounce or force stretches. If, for example, your leg starts to shake as you stretch it, you have pushed it too far. You should feel the tension, but there should not be any pain.

■ If you work at a computer screen, have it positioned directly in front of you and have your chair adjusted to the correct height.

Take Care

These exercises are not intended for those suffering from chronic back pain. Prior to starting them, see your doctor or a back specialist for advice. If any of these exercises causes pain, then stop immediately.

Soothing PMS

Gentle, soothing exercise, acupressure, and relaxation work wonders on premenstrual syndrome (PMS) symptoms. These gentle exercises improve your circulation, carrying blood and oxygen to the relevant muscles, helping to relieve cramps related to your period. They can also help relieve bloating and backache, and even lift your mood making you feel less irritable. Before reaching for the pain killers, stretch out instead. You will need towels, pillows, and a wall for support.

REDUCE BLOATING

Stack two folded towels against a wall and lie with your buttocks on top of the towels, your legs against the wall, with a towel under your head and shoulders. Position a rolled-up towel under your neck. Try to get your legs as upright as possible, but don't worry if they are at an angle to the wall. Rest the heel and palms of your hands on your hip bones. Press your fingers gently but firmly into the fold of the skin where the thigh and the hip meet for around 30 seconds. Breathe deeply. Relax for a few minutes.

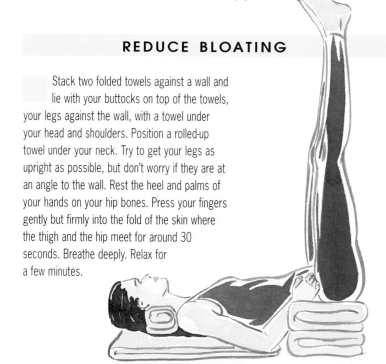

RELIEVE CRAMPS

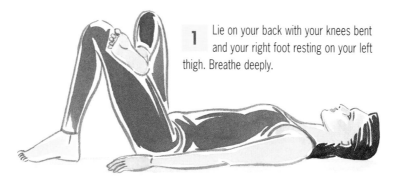

1 Lie on your back with your knees bent and your right foot resting on your left thigh. Breathe deeply.

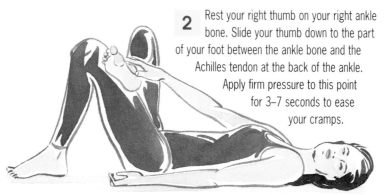

2 Rest your right thumb on your right ankle bone. Slide your thumb down to the part of your foot between the ankle bone and the Achilles tendon at the back of the ankle. Apply firm pressure to this point for 3–7 seconds to ease your cramps.

EASE BACKACHE

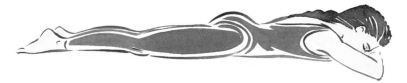

Lie flat on your stomach with your toes touching and your heels falling comfortably apart. Place your palms flat, one on top of the other, and rest your forehead on them. Close your eyes and inhale, pressing your abdomen deep down into the floor, tightening your buttocks. Breathe out as you relax. Repeat as often as you like.

HELPFUL HEALTH TIPS

■ Chamomile tea can help to relieve menstrual cramps and has a sedative effect to relax you. Let this herbal tea "brew" for 10 minutes before drinking to get the full effect.

■ Avoid sugary and refined carbohydrate foods, such as cakes and cookies, even if your body appears to crave them. Try eating small carbohydrate snacks, such as crackers or crispbreads, regularly throughout the day instead.

■ Exercise releases natural pain killers, called endorphins. Try going for a swim if your cramps are not too severe.

■ Warmth can ease cramps, so try a warm aromatherapy bath (see page 88). Sweet marjoram essential oil in the bath or in an aromatherapy diffuser is helpful.

3

EatWell

Healthy Eating **Is Key** to looking and feeling good. **A well-balanced diet can help to keep your energy reserves constant—after you eat a chocolate bar you'll get a surge of energy, followed by a sudden dip; eating a banana, which releases its energy slowly and constantly, will keep your hunger at bay for much longer. Choosing the right foods can also prevent disease and keep your weight down. Best of all, good, fresh food doesn't need to be time-consuming, expensive, or hard to prepare, as you'll see from the ideas and recipes contained in this section.**

FUEL You may feel fine for a short period of time living on convenience and junk foods, but the quality of the nutrition you will be getting is poor. Sooner or later, you'll notice a deterioration in your health—lower energy levels, poorer complexion and dull hair, greater tendency to catch colds. In the long term, your body will run most effectively on the best fuel, just as cars do. What exactly makes the best food fuel is not always clear, especially when the experts seem to change their minds almost daily about whether margarine is healthier than butter, eggs are good or bad for you, or red wine is better than white. There is one thing that nutritionists are universally agreed upon, and that is that the healthiest diet is low in fat

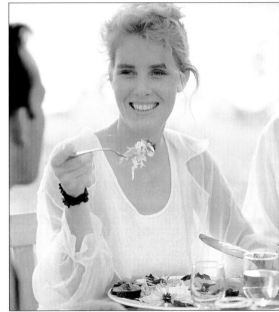

PLAN and cholesterol, low in sodium and refined sugar, high in fiber and complex carbohydrates, and packed with vitamin-rich fruit and vegetables.

Most people know these principles, but eating healthily sometimes seems too much of a chore. We eat whatever is available: convenience food, junk food, take-out. As we get older, we feel the effects of this kind of diet—we put on weight, feel more lethargic, and look less healthy. Eating well need not be time-consuming, tedious, and tasteless—it's a matter of getting into good habits and making good food choices. Try to plan ahead, make use of the healthier packaged foods, select a wide range of ingredients, and use plenty of flavorings, such as herbs and spices.

BALANCE It's thought that certain foods can boost energy levels, make you sleep better, boost the immune system, possibly even ward off cancer and osteoporosis. By understanding which nutrients make you feel good, give you maximum energy, and protect your body from disease, you can fuel your body with everything it needs to keep it running smoothly and efficiently. You'll find healthy food can taste good too!

Read&Digest

A balanced diet means eating a variety of food from the main food groups. By choosing from these categories you ensure that your body gets all the nutrients and energy it needs. As a guide, carbohydrates should provide about 55–60 percent of your energy needs, protein around 5–10 percent, fats 30 percent or less. Less than than 10 percent of calories should be from saturated fat.

The problem in the West is that we tend to eat too much fat and refined (processed) carbohydrates, especially sugar. To achieve the healthiest diet, choose foods low in fat, sodium, and sugar, but high in minerals, vitamins, fiber and complex carbohydrates.

IT'S ALL IN A DAY'S FOOD

Breakfast

Ideally breakfast should be the biggest meal of the day, lunch moderate and dinner light. Half a grapefruit (or fruit juice), cereal such as oatmeal or bran flakes, and a slice of whole wheat toast without butter are nutrient-rich choices. The grapefruit is full of vitamin C, the milk full of calcium, the cereal loaded with vitamins and fiber, the toast full of fiber and complex carbohydrate. Try to make low-fat, low-sugar foods a way of life for all the family.

Lunch

Make time to eat lunch because it will provide you with the energy (physical and mental) to carry on through the afternoon. A good example of an easy-to-prepare lunch is a homemade vegetable soup that is low in fat and high in protein, and chicken with mixed greens on sliced whole wheat bread. This will supply you with protein, essential B vitamins, other vitamins, minerals, fiber, and unrefined carbohydrate. To flavor the sandwich, choose pepper and lemon juice instead of salt, butter, and mayonnaise.

Dinner

Broiled fish or skinless chicken with rice and vegetables is a well-balanced meal with protein, vitamins, minerals, carbohydrate, and fiber. Cooking the fish or chicken in just a little oil with lemon juice and fresh herbs keeps it low in fat and full of flavor. A fresh fruit salad or yogurt makes a low-fat dessert.

Take Care

Alcohol in excess does not have any health benefits, but the occasional glass of wine or beer may reduce the risk of heart disease. Many health organizations and nutrition experts recommend moderation in consumption of alcohol. Most guidelines suggest that you limit your intake to 2 drinks per day. One drink consists of 8–12 fl oz/ 250–375 ml beer, 2 tbsp/30 ml hard liquor, or 3–4 fl oz/90–125 ml wine.

DAILY INTAKE OF FOOD GROUPS

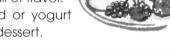

FATS,
OILS &
SUGARS
Use sparingly

2–3 servings: eg. 1 cup (250 ml) milk, 2 oz (50 g) cheese, ¾ cup (175 g) yogurt.

MILK, CHEESE & YOGURT

FISH, MEAT, POULTRY, EGGS, NUTS & DRY BEANS

2–3 servings: eg. 2–3½ oz (50–100 g) fish, meat, poultry, 2 eggs, 2 tbsp peanut butter, 1 cup (250 g) beans.

VEGETABLES
3–5 servings: eg. 1 medium-size, 1 cup raw, or ½ cup cooked vegetables, ½ cup juice.

FRUIT
2–4 servings: eg. 1 medium-size fruit, ½ cup fresh fruit juice.

BREAD, CEREAL, RICE & PASTA
6–10 servings: eg. 1 slice bread, ½ bagel or pita, half cup pasta or rice. Choose whole wheat often.

To minimize the fat content of your diet (see Fat Facts on page 54), select low-fat (skim) milk, and low-fat cheese and yogurt, whenever possible. Look for lean cuts of meat, and remove the skin from poultry prior to cooking. To maximize your intake of the antioxidant vitamins C and A (as betacarotene) eat fresh, dark green and orange vegetables often (see page 78).

In Canada, the recommended daily intake of food groups is:
Fat, oils & sugars—use sparingly
Milk, cheese & yogurt—2–4 servings
Fish, meat, poultry, eggs, nuts & dry beans—2–3 servings
Vegetables & fruit—5–10 servings
Bread, cereals, rice & pasta—5–12 servings

WaysToStaySlim

Losing weight and keeping it off can be achieved by making relatively small changes to your lifestyle. You can stay slim for life without missing out on the foods you enjoy, but you may need to moderate your consumption of them. For an ideal weight and good health choose a variety of low-fat, low-sugar foods and exercise regularly. Follow the advice below for a slimmer, more healthy future.

TEN SIMPLE SLIMMING SECRETS

1 Think positive
Don't think in terms of denial and punishment when trying to lose weight or maintain weight loss. Think instead of long-term healthier eating, better health, and a better-looking you.

2 Balance your body's needs
There is no big secret about losing weight. If your intake of calories exceeds your body's needs, you gain weight. It pays to be realistic about how much you eat and what you eat.

3 Measure it!
Weigh food portions to get an idea of what a recommended serving looks like —it's smaller than you think! Don't eat foods, such as ice cream or yogurt, straight out of the carton, instead measure out a portion.

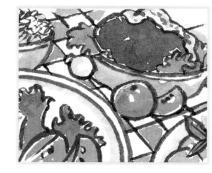

4 Ban buffets
You don't have to stop eating out, but do think about what you're eating and where. For example, you're more likely to lose track of how much you're eating at an "Eat as Much as You Like" buffet than at a sit-down dinner. The golden rule is to avoid anything fried, fatty, or creamy. Beware of "hidden" fats. Chicken, for example, is lean, but the skin is not.

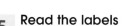

5 Read the labels
Always read the food labels to check for fat and sugar content. Try to use low-calorie products —you will soon find that the higher-fat and sugar varieties taste too rich. Beware, some low-fat products contain a lot of sugar, which will add to your calorie intake.

6 Weigh yourself weekly
Don't keep weighing yourself. If you are on a weight-loss diet, jump on the scales every week or so but don't become fanatical. Weight can fluctuate during your monthly hormonal cycle.

7 Take water with your wine
You don't have to give up alcohol when you're trying to lose weight, but you do need to cut down and stick to lower-calorie drinks, such as dry white wine, clear spirits, and fruit-based cocktails, instead of beers and creamy cocktails. Stick to low-calorie mixers, and follow every alcoholic drink with a large glass of mineral water.

8 Eat regular meals
Don't skip meals and do aim for a realistic weight loss. If you skip meals to lose weight quickly, you are more likely to disrupt your metabolism and ultimately put weight back on. Aim to lose 1–2 lb (500 g–1 kg) per week.

9 Exercise to lose weight faster
To lose weight faster, cut down on your calorie consumption and take regular exercise.

10 Cut out convenience foods
There are very few low-fat or healthy fast foods—so try to cut them out. Avoid convenience foods too because they are often high in fats and sodium to enhance their flavor.

FatFacts

We need to carry a certain amount of fat on our bodies—it's the body's form of stored energy and helps keep us warm! We can, of course, store too much fat and dietary fat is the food most easily converted to body fat. Health guidelines suggest we should get no more than 30 percent of our daily calorie intake from fat, and only 10 percent or less coming from saturated fat. This will control your weight and reduce the risk of heart disease and some cancers. All fats provide 9 calories per gram, about twice as many calories as carbohydrate or protein.

TEN WAYS TO CUT DOWN ON FATS

1 Moderate your fat intake
Fat should make up one-third of your calorie intake, and one-third of that can be saturated fats such as animal fats. This isn't based solely on the amount of food—a portion of cheese has twice as many calories as the same weight of pasta.

2 Look after your heart
Cut down on saturated fats. As well as reducing calories, a diet low in animal fats and rich in olive oil may lower the risk of heart disease. Use margarine made with olive oil and avoid hydrogenated margarine, which is also linked to heart disease.

3 Read labels carefully
Read nutrition labels carefully, many products that are labeled reduced fat or light may still be high in calories, sodium, or fat. Whenever possible choose foods marked fat-free (less than 0.5 g of fat per serving), or low-fat (3 g of fat or less per serving).

4 Get mean with meat
Trim off excess fat from meat. Buy leaner cuts of red meat and ground beef. Try alternatives such as skinless poultry, soya, tofu, or white fish.

5 Down with dairy
Use low-fat alternatives to products such as cream, mayonnaise, yogurt, and cheese. Substitute fat-free or low-fat milk (skim) for whole milk.

6 Use yogurt
Serve low-fat frozen yogurt instead of ice cream for dessert. If you can't live without ice cream, try a half ice cream, half frozen yogurt combination. Mix plain yogurt with sour cream to put on baked potatoes.

7 Spray or sauté
Use non-stick cooking spray instead of oil. Alternatively, "sauté" onions and other basic sauce ingredients in reduced sodium stock.

8 Finish with frying
Steam, stir-fry, dry fry (without oil), broil, or bake when possible instead of frying food in oil. If a recipe calls for oil, use olive oil wherever possible.

9 Keep salads simple
Creamy dressings, such as blue cheese or Caesar, are high in calories. Try fat-free alternatives. At a restaurant, ask for dressing on the side so you can monitor how much you use.

10 Watch out for hidden fat
Convenience foods use fats to enhance the flavor, so cut down on cookies, chocolate, pastries, and potato chips.

Where to Find Fat

SATURATED FATS
Foods high in saturated fat can raise blood cholesterol levels which subsequently clogs blood vessels, increasing the risk of coronary heart disease. Found in red meat • egg yolk • cheese • fats solid at room temperature, such as butter and lard • whole milk • ice cream • coconut oil • palm oil.

UNSATURATED FATS
Polyunsaturated
Found in most oils, such as soybean, corn, sunflower, cottonseed, safflower • walnuts • almonds • oily fish such as salmon, tuna, herring, swordfish, mackerel. These fish also contain fatty acids known to lower cholesterol.

Monounsaturated
Found in olive oil, which also helps drive down cholesterol levels • canola oil • avocado oil.

Vital Vitamins

Without the recommended daily intake of vitamins, your health can suffer. Your diet should provide most of them, but if you have been ill, are not eating a balanced diet, have been skipping meals, eating too much overprocessed food, or have special nutritional needs (if you're anemic or pregnant), you may require vitamin supplements, especially vitamins A, C, and E. These are antioxidants which help protect against the damage to cells and tissues caused by free radicals. Take 10 minutes to study this guide to see if your daily diet contains all the vitamins you need.

AT-A-GLANCE GUIDE TO VITAMINS

■ Vitamin A
Found in liver, egg yolk, milk products. Retinol, a form of vitamin A, is made from the betacarotene found in green, leafy vegetables like broccoli, and yellow-orange fruit and vegetables like sweet potatoes, carrots, mango.
Function: Maintains healthy skin and hair, forms bones and teeth during childhood, functions in the development and maintenance of the linings of respiratory, digestive, and urinary tracts, maintains night vision.

■ Vitamin B1 (thiamine)
Found in whole wheat bread, brown rice, pasta, whole grain cereals, bran, liver, kidney, fish, peas, nuts, beans, eggs, green vegetables like collard greens.
Function: Essential for releasing energy from food, and normal nerve function.

■ Vitamin B2 (riboflavin)
Found in milk, liver, eggs, cheese, green vegetables, brewer's yeast, whole grains, wheat germ.
Function: Essential for releasing energy from food, promotes production of hormones by the adrenal glands, maintains healthy mouth, tongue, and skin, and formation of red blood cells.

■ Vitamin B3 (niacin)
Found in lean meats, poultry, fish, nuts, dried beans.
Function: Essential for releasing energy from carbohydrates, promotes the production of hormones and the formation of red blood cells.

■ Vitamin B6 (pyridoxine)
Found in liver, poultry, pork, fish, potatoes, dried beans, most dried fruits, avocados, cabbage, cauliflower, soybeans, nuts, brewer's yeast, whole wheat bread, whole grain cereals.
Function: Helps maintain healthy blood cells and nervous system, helps release energy from food.

■ Vitamin B12
Found only in products of animal origin such as poultry, liver, pork, fish, yeast, eggs, dairy products. (Vegetarians are advised to take this as a supplement.)
Function: Essential for formation of red and white blood cells, helps keep the nervous system healthy.

■ Folic acid
Found in leafy green vegetables, oranges, liver, nuts, whole wheat bread.
Function: Formation of blood cells, essential for women who are trying to conceive or who are pregnant, to ensure healthy development of the fetus.

■ Vitamin C
Found in fruit and vegetables.
Function: Helps maintain healthy gums, teeth, bones, and blood vessels, a healthy immune system, enhances wound healing, helps iron absorption.

■ Vitamin D
Found in oily fish, milk, liver, egg yolk, cod-liver oil and other fish oils, fortified cereals. It is added to some margarines.
Function: Formation and maintenance of bones and teeth, and absorption of calcium.

■ Vitamin E
Found in vegetable oils, margarine, nuts, whole grain cereals, whole wheat bread, dried beans, green leafy vegetables.
Function: Promoting formation of new blood cells, protecting cells from damage and aging.

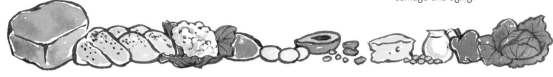

HELPFUL HEALTH TIPS

■ Buying ready-prepared, pre-peeled, and sliced vegetables might seem like a good time-saving idea but the cut surfaces actually lose vitamins. Frozen vegetables, which are quickly frozen after picking, can contain more vitamins than fresh produce that has been hanging around losing valuable vitamin and mineral content.

■ Steam or stir-fry rather than boil vegetables. Valuable vitamins, especially vitamin C, can be lost in boiling. If you do boil vegetables, use just a little water and cook them very lightly. Keep the water for making stock for other recipes.

■ Try to eat as many raw vegetables as you can to maximize your vitamin intake. Water soluble vitamins, such as C and B complex, are easily lost as they dissolve in boiling water during cooking.

Cold Breakfasts

Having a nutrient-rich food or drink for breakfast is a fast way of boosting your energy levels and making you healthier. You use up around 600 calories just sleeping, and if you don't eat breakfast, your blood-sugar levels drop off by mid-morning. This makes you lethargic, reduces your ability to concentrate, and makes you more likely to reach for something sweet or fatty to fill you up and give you instant energy. Try eating these low-fat, high-energy breakfasts for a month and see if you don't perform better. Try these breakfasts when you've little time to spare or during the summer months when cold breakfasts are more appealing.

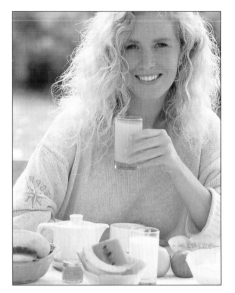

OATMEAL MUESLI

You will need: *2 tbsp oat bran, 4 tbsp rolled oats, 4 tbsp/60 ml low-fat plain yogurt, fat-free milk, 1 tbsp pumpkin seeds, ½ sliced banana, a few dried figs or apricots (optional)* **Serves 1**

1 Mix the oat bran, rolled oats, and yogurt together, adding some fat-free milk if too thick. Cover the mixture with plastic food wrap and refrigerate overnight.
2 Mix in the seeds and top with the fruit. Add extra fat-free milk if required.

FRUITY FLAKES

You will need: *¾ cup/1½ oz/45 g bran flakes, 1 peach, a few strawberries, fat-free milk to serve* **Serves 1**

1 Top the bran flakes with the pitted, sliced peach and halved strawberries. Serve with fat-free milk.

DRIED FRUIT YOGURT

You will need: *1 cup/4 oz/125 g dried fruit salad, ⅔ cup/5 fl oz/150 ml low-fat plain yogurt, pinch ground cinnamon, 1 tbsp/15 ml clear honey, 1 tbsp pumpkin seeds* **Serves 1**

1 Snip the fruit into small pieces with scissors. Stir the fruit into the yogurt with the cinnamon and honey. Scatter the pumpkin seeds over the top before serving.

BANANA & CINNAMON BAGELS

You will need: *1 cinnamon and raisin bagel, 1 banana, 2 tbsp/30 ml fromage frais or low-fat yogurt, 1 tbsp/15 ml maple syrup* **Serves 1**

1 Halve the bagel and toast inside. Top with the sliced banana and the fromage frais or yogurt. Drizzle over the maple syrup before serving.

STRAWBERRY SURPRISE

You will need: *4 oz/125 g strawberries, ½ cup/ 4 fl oz/125 ml low-fat plain yogurt, 1 tsp/5 ml clear honey, 1 tbsp toasted sunflower seeds* **Serves 1**

1 Halve the strawberries and place in a bowl. Top with the yogurt. Drizzle over the honey and top with the sunflower seeds.

FRUIT WITH MAPLE CHEESE

You will need: *1½ cups/12 fl oz/375 ml ready-prepared exotic fruit salad, 4 tbsp/60 ml fromage frais or low-fat yogurt, 1 tbsp/15 ml maple syrup, 1 tsp toasted shredded coconut* **Serves 1**

1 Put the fruit salad in a bowl. Spoon over the fromage frais or yogurt and maple syrup. Scatter the coconut over the top before serving.

Hot Breakfasts

When the temperature outside drops, one of these warming breakfasts will help you start the day full of energy.

BREAKFAST OMELET

You will need: *¼ sweet red pepper, 2 green onions, 1 tomato, 2 eggs or egg substitute, 1 tbsp/15 ml water, 1 tsp chopped parsley, non-stick spray, 1 slice whole wheat toast* **Serves 1**

1 Sauté the pepper, green onions, and tomato in a non-stick omelet pan for 5 minutes.
2 Whisk the eggs and water with plenty of ground black pepper. Add the eggs and parsley to the pan and cook, stirring occasionally, until the egg has set. Serve with the whole wheat toast.

WARM FRUITY OATMEAL

You will need: *¾ cup/1½ oz/40 g rolled oats, ⅔ cup/5 fl oz/ 150 ml fat-free milk, ⅔ cup/5 fl oz/150 ml water, ½ sliced banana, 6 chopped dried apricots* **Serves 1**

1 Put the oats, milk, and water into a saucepan and slowly bring to a boil, stirring occasionally. Simmer gently until thickened.
2 Stir in the fruit and let stand for 5 minutes before serving.

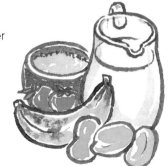

BANANA TOASTS

You will need: *2 slices whole wheat bread, 1 banana, 2 tsp/10 ml maple syrup, pinch grated nutmeg, 2 tsp sesame seeds* **Serves 1**

1 Toast the bread on one side only under the broiler.
2 Mash the banana and spread onto the untoasted side of the whole wheat toast. Drizzle over the maple syrup and scatter sesame seeds on top. Return to the broiler until the seeds are golden.

SMOKED FISH SCRAMBLE

You will need: *1 bagel, 1 large egg or egg substitute, 2 tbsp/30 ml cottage cheese, 1 oz/30 g smoked trout or lox, 1 tsp snipped chives, freshly ground black pepper* **Serves 1**

1 Warm the bagel. Meanwhile put the egg in a saucepan and beat while heating gently. When the egg has scrambled, stir in the cottage cheese, smoked trout, chives, and plenty of black pepper.
2 Halve the bagel and top with the egg scramble.

EGG & BACON CAKES

You will need: *1 potato cake, 2 strips lean bacon, 1 small egg or egg substitute, a few fresh parsley leaves* **Serves 1**

1 Toast the potato cake on both sides. Broil the bacon until crisp, and crumble. Poach the egg for 3 minutes in a saucepan of boiling water.
2 Top the toasted potato cake with the egg and bacon. Scatter the parsley leaves over the egg and serve.

HealthFruit Juices

Drinking fresh fruit and vegetable juices is a quick way to add vitamins and minerals to your diet. A juice makes an easy, nutritious light meal or a great between-meals snack. Homemade fruit juices can be kept fresh in the refrigerator for up to 24 hours, but try to drink them as soon as you can as they soon lose a great deal of their valuable vitamin and mineral content.

LIQUID BREAKFAST

You will need: *4 oz/125 g banana (or strawberries, peach, pineapple, or mango), 1¼ cups/½ pint/300 ml fat-free milk, 1 tsp/5 ml clear honey, 1 tsp sesame seeds* **Serves 1**

1 Peel the bananas, or the fruit of your choice, and chop.
2 Place the fruit in a blender and add the milk and honey. Blend until smooth, pour into a glass, and top with the sesame seeds.

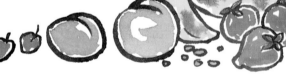

SPICED ORCHARD DRINK

You will need: *2 apples, 1 pear, juice of ½ lemon, pinch ground cinnamon, ½ cup/4 fl oz/125 ml mineral water* **Serves 1**

1 Peel (optional) and core the fruit and blend in a blender with the remaining ingredients until smooth.
2 Pass through a coarse sieve, pour into a glass, and serve.

EXOTIC CRUSH

You will need: *1 small ripe mango, 1 small pawpaw, 1 passion fruit, ½ banana, ½ cup/4 fl oz/ 125 ml fat-free milk* **Serves 1**

1 Peel, deseed, and chop the mango and pawpaw. Place in a blender with the passion fruit pulp, banana, and milk.
2 Blend together until smooth. Pour into a glass to serve.

STRAWBERRY DAWN

You will need: *4 oz/125 g strawberries, ⅔ cup/5 fl oz/150 ml low-fat strawberry yogurt, juice of ½ lime, 1 tsp/5 ml clear honey, fat-free milk* **Serves 1**

1 Blend together the strawberries, yogurt, lime juice, and honey until smooth.
2 Pour into a glass and top up with the fat-free milk. Stir well and serve.

ENERGY BOOSTER JUICE

You will need: *1 small mango, ¼ pineapple, 1 banana, ½ cup/4 fl oz/ 125 ml fat-free milk, ¼ cup/2 fl oz/ 50 ml plain yogurt, ½ tsp shredded coconut, 1 tsp/5 ml clear honey, a few sesame seeds* **Serves 1**

1 Peel and chop the mango, pineapple, and banana. Place in a blender, blend until smooth, and pour into a jar.
2 Add the remaining ingredients and stir.

CITRUS ZINGER

You will need: *1 orange, 1 grapefruit, ½ lime, ½-in/1-cm cube of fresh ginger, sparkling mineral water (optional)* **Serves 1**

1 Squeeze the juices from the citrus fruit and pour into a glass. Peel and finely grate the ginger and squeeze the juice (about ¼ tsp/1.5 ml) into the glass. Discard the remaining ginger pulp.
2 Top up with mineral water (optional) and serve.

Vegetable Juices

Fresh vegetable juices, like fruit juices, are quick to prepare, packed with vitamins and minerals, and a good way of boosting your consumption of raw vegetables. Vegetable juices can be an acquired taste, so if they are new to you, start with Carrot Crush—a delicious blend of fruit and vegetable.

GAZPACHO IN A GLASS

You will need: *1 small sweet red pepper, ½ cucumber, 4 tomatoes, small handful watercress, sparkling mineral water* **Serves 1**

1 Remove seeds from the pepper. Roughly chop the pepper, cucumber, and tomatoes and place in a blender with the watercress. Blend until smooth.
2 Pour into a glass and top up with mineral water, add a pinch of sea salt, and freshly ground black pepper. Stir well and serve.

CARROT CRUSH

You will need: *3 carrots, juice of 1 orange, 6 tbsp/3 fl oz/90 ml mineral water* **Serves 1**

1 Finely grate the carrots in a food processor. Add the orange juice and water, then blend until smooth.
2 Pour through a coarse sieve and squeeze the juice out into a bowl. Pour into a glass and serve.

MINTY CUCUMBER COOLER

You will need: *½ cucumber, small handful fresh mint leaves, juice of ½ lime, 6 tbsp/3 fl oz/90 ml mineral water* **Serves 1**

1 Chop the cucumber and place in a blender with the mint, lime juice, and mineral water.
2 Blend together until smooth. Pour into a glass and serve.

BEET BREAK

You will need: *2 large raw beets, juice of ½ lemon, 2 stalks celery* **Serves 1**

1 Peel and finely grate the beets with the grater attachment of a food processor. Add the lemon and chopped celery, and blend together until smooth.
2 Pour through a sieve into a bowl. Pour into a glass and serve.

Take Care

Juicing can give you many of the vitamins and minerals you need, but not the fiber. So, if you prefer your juices sieved, ensure you eat whole fruit and vegetables too. Juices should not be seen as a substitute. Some juicing advocates suggest an occasional day's fast— drinking only juices and mineral water. Although this may not be harmful, doctors caution that it could deprive your body of energy and a balance of nutrients.

HELPFUL HEALTH TIPS

■ Whenever possible, use organic fruit and vegetables for juicing.

■ Serve any of the fruit juices as a healthy dessert. It's a great way to satisfy a sweet-tooth craving.

■ Some people claim to find particular fruit or vegetable juice combinations helpful in easing certain conditions:
insomnia—celery, lettuce, watercress, grapefruit, raspberry;
PMS—sweet peppers, leeks, carrot, apple, blackberry;
stress—blackcurrant, citrus fruit, green leafy vegetables, apricot, avocado, melon;
water retention—carrot, celery, cucumber, parsley, cranberry, apple, pineapple.

Fix-ahead Snacks

When you feel hunger pangs between meals, try to keep the principles of healthy eating firmly in mind. It's all too easy to let good intentions slip when potato chips and candy are on hand. Stock your shelves with foods that are low in fat and sugar and high in fiber. When you have time, make up some fix-

ahead snacks. The three basic recipes here can be adapted in various ways to provide a wide array of quick, healthy fillers. While hummus needs to be refrigerated, the Exotic Dried Fruit Mix and Spicy Popcorn are ideal snacking foods that can go with you anywhere. Keep a small jar in the office, or in your backpack when out walking.

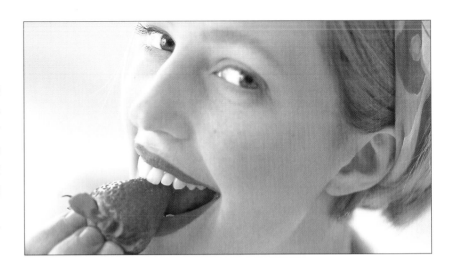

BASIC HUMMUS

You will need: 2 tbsp toasted sesame seeds, 2 cans (15½ oz/420 g) chick peas, 2 large garlic cloves, juice of ½ lemon, 2 tbsp chopped parsley **Serves 4**

1 Place all the ingredients except the parsley in a blender, plus 4 tbsp/60 ml of liquid from the chick peas. Blend until smooth and creamy.
2 Stir in the parsley before serving. Keep refrigerated—it will stay fresh for up to 3 days.

Variations:
- Cook a potato in the microwave and top with hummus.
- Serve with raw vegetables.
- Toss into pasta with a little vegetable broth.
- Serve with warm whole wheat pita rounds.
- Spoon into pita rounds with chopped, cooked chicken, lettuce, and tomatoes.

EXOTIC DRIED FRUIT MIX

You will need: 3 tbsp dried, shredded coconut, 3 tbsp pumpkin seeds, 4 oz/125 g each dried figs, apricots, mango, pears, and peaches **Serves 4**

1 Spread the coconut and pumpkin seeds on a baking sheet and toast until golden.
2 Combine the coconut and pumpkin seeds with the fruit and let cool. Store in an airtight container. It will keep fresh for up to a month.

Variations:
- Finely chop some Exotic Dried Fruit Mix and stir into plain yogurt with a little honey.
- Stir some Exotic Dried Fruit Mix into cooked rice and toss in fat-free vinaigrette while still warm.
- Add Exotic Dried Fruit Mix to grated carrots. Toss with fat-free vinaigrette dressing for an instant salad.

SPICY POPCORN

You will need: 2 tsp/10 ml corn oil, ¼ tsp ground cumin, ¼ tsp ground coriander, ¼ tsp paprika, 5 tbsp popcorn kernels **Serves 4**

1 Heat the oil in a large saucepan. Add the spices, then the popcorn kernels. Cover tightly and cook over a moderate heat for 5 minutes, shaking the saucepan frequently until the popping stops.
2 Serve immediately with a little cracked salt, or let cool and pack in an airtight container.

Variations:
- Omit the spices and drizzle a little honey over the popcorn just before eating.
- Chop some fresh parsley and chives and add to the warm popcorn.
- Mix some sweet chili sauce and a little dark soy sauce, and drizzle over the warm popcorn. Toss well and eat immediately.

Speedy Snacks

These quick-to-prepare snack recipes can be real life-savers when hunger hits you. They are tasty, and will see you through a low-energy time. If time is even too short for these, look to the Tips column for store-bought items that can be good substitutes!

MINI PIZZAS

You will need: 1 English muffin, 2 tbsp mixed pepper antipasto or canned pimiento, sliced, 1 sliced tomato, 4 slices low-fat mozzarella cheese, shredded basil leaves **Serves 1**

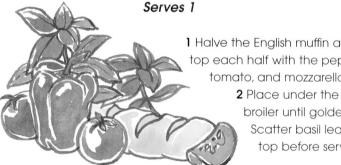

1 Halve the English muffin and top each half with the peppers, tomato, and mozzarella.
2 Place under the broiler until golden. Scatter basil leaves on top before serving.

CUCUMBER DIP WITH CRUDITÉS

You will need: ⅔ cup/5 fl oz/150 ml low-fat plain yogurt, ¼ cucumber, grated, 1 small garlic clove, crushed, handful fresh mint, chopped vegetable strips (such as carrot, celery, and sweet pepper) **Serves 1**

1 Mix together the yogurt, drained cucumber, garlic, and mint and spoon into a bowl.
2 Serve with vegetable strips.

SMOKED FISH PÂTÉ

You will need: 4 oz/120 g smoked mackerel fillet, 1 green onion, 3 tbsp/45 ml low-fat crème fraîche or low-fat sour cream, 1 tsp/5 ml creamed horseradish, squeeze lemon juice, whole wheat toast to serve **Serves 1**

1 Flake the fish into a blender and add the rest of the ingredients. Blend until smooth.
2 Serve with whole wheat toast.

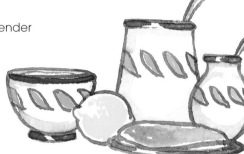

GOAT CHEESE TOASTS

You will need: 2 slices French bread, 1 garlic clove, 4 slices low-fat goat cheese **Serves 1**

1 Toast both sides of the bread. Cut the garlic clove in half and rub all over the toast.
2 Top with the slices of cheese, and return to the broiler until golden.

COTTAGE CHEESE ON RYE

You will need: 1 slice light rye bread, 2 tbsp/30 ml low-fat cottage cheese, handful mixed lettuce, 3 cherry tomatoes, 1 tsp/5 ml fat-free vinaigrette dressing, ground black pepper **Serves 1**

1 Spread the rye bread with the cottage cheese. Top with the lettuce leaves and tomatoes, and drizzle over some fat-free vinaigrette dressing. Grind black pepper on top.

HELPFUL HEALTH TIPS

■ Go for energy-boosting ingredients—apricots (dried or fresh); figs (dried or fresh); bananas; buckwheat; maize; oats; wheat; wheat germ; most nuts; seeds; most vegetables and fruits; complex carbohydrates (grains and legumes). These gradually release sugar into the bloodstream. If you are trying to lose weight moderate your intake of dried fruits—as they are high in sugar as well as beneficial fiber, vitamins, and minerals—and nuts and seeds, which are high in fat.

■ Stock up on these instant snacks—mixed light raisins, dark raisins, and sunflower seeds; bagels; rice cakes; plain yogurt; unsweetened breakfast cereals (eat them any time of day); vegetable strips kept in the refrigerator.

Packed Lunches 1

Lunch is an all-important meal. If you miss it, your energy levels will slump in the afternoon making you feel exhausted and your mind "fuzzy." This doesn't mean that you should indulge in a three-course feast, as over-eating at midday can make you just as tired as not eating at all. For high energy in the afternoon, go for one of these low-fat lunches. They can be prepacked and stored in the refrigerator, and are tasty and nutritious. What's more—they can be made in less than 10 minutes.

RUSTIC TUNA ROLL

You will need: *1 rustic roll, 2 tbsp/30 ml fat-free vinaigrette dressing, 1 tomato, 1 can (3 oz/90 g) tuna in spring water, 1 tsp capers, 1 tbsp fresh chopped basil, a handful fresh greens (lettuce or arugula)* **Serves 1**

1 Split the roll and hollow out some of the middle. Drizzle a little of the dressing inside the roll and fill with tomato slices.
2 Mix the tuna, capers, and basil together with the remaining dressing and a little seasoning.
3 Spoon the tuna into the roll, top with greens and the bread lid. Cover with plastic food wrap and store in the refrigerator.

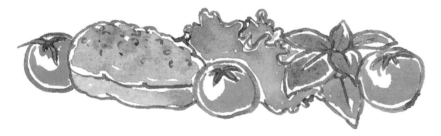

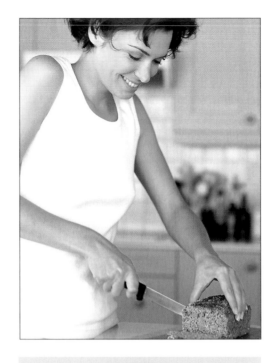

TLT

You will need: *2 thick slices whole-grain bread, 1 tbsp/15 ml low-fat mayonnaise, 4 oz/125 g smoked tofu or smoked turkey, handful of shredded mixed lettuce leaves, 1 tomato, ½ small sweet red onion* **Serves 1**

1 Spread one slice of the bread with mayonnaise and top with slices of smoked tofu or smoked turkey, lettuce, tomato, and thin slices of onion.
2 Season with black pepper and top with the other bread slice. Cover with plastic food wrap and store in the refrigerator.

CRUNCHY TURKEY MIX

You will need: *2 oz/60 g light cream cheese, 1 tbsp/15 ml fat-free milk, ½ red apple, 1 stalk celery, a few seedless purple grapes, 1 whole wheat pita round, handful mixed greens, 1 oz/30 g wafer-thin smoked turkey* **Serves 1**

1 Mix the cream cheese and milk together until smooth. Stir in finely chopped apple, sliced celery, and purple grapes.
2 Pile into the pita round and top with the greens, turkey, and plenty of ground black pepper. Cover with plastic food wrap and store in the refrigerator.

LEMON SHRIMP IN SEEDED BREAD

You will need: *2 slices mixed seed bread, 1 tbsp/ 15 ml low-fat mayonnaise, 2 oz/60 g cooked, shelled, and deveined shrimp, handful mixed fresh greens and herbs, 1 tomato, squeeze fresh lemon juice* **Serves 1**

1 Spread the bread with the mayonnaise and top with the shrimp, greens and herbs, sliced tomato, and lemon juice.
2 Add plenty of black pepper and top with the remaining slice of bread. Cover with plastic food wrap and store in the refrigerator.

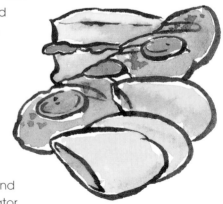

PackedLunches2

Be adventurous with sandwich fillings. Look out for goat cheese, chicken tikka or smoked chicken—their unique flavor will add a lift to your packed lunch. It's wise only to eat some of the following ingredients in moderation. For example, shrimp is high in cholesterol, while ham is often high in sodium.

GOAT CHEESE & PEPPER BAGUETTES

You will need: *1 small baguette, 4 tbsp/60 ml low-fat goat cheese, 1 green onion, 2 tbsp/30 ml mixed pepper antipasto or canned pimiento, sliced, a few fresh thyme leaves* **Serves 1**

1 Split the baguette and spread the goat cheese inside.
2 Top with finely chopped green onion, mixed pepper antipasto or pimiento, thyme leaves, and plenty of ground black pepper. Cover with plastic food wrap and store in the refrigerator.

INDIAN PITA POCKET

You will need: *4 oz/125 g precooked chicken tikka or barbecued chicken, 2 tbsp/30 ml low-fat crème fraîche or low-fat sour cream, squeeze lemon juice, 1 tbsp cilantro leaves, handful finely shredded lettuce, cucumber slices, 1 whole wheat pita round* **Serves 1**

1 Chop the chicken and stir into the crème fraîche or sour cream.
2 Toss the lemon juice into the cilantro, lettuce, and cucumber.
3 Split open the pita and fill with the lettuce mixture. Top with the chicken. Cover in plastic food wrap and store in the refrigerator.

SMOKED CHICKEN CLUB SANDWICH

You will need: *2 thin slices whole wheat toast, 2 tbsp/30 ml low-fat mayonnaise, 2 slices smoked chicken, 1 tomato, handful watercress* **Serves 1**

1 Spread one slice of toast with mayonnaise and top with the chicken, tomato, and watercress. Top with the remaining slice.
2 Add plenty of freshly ground black pepper. Cover with plastic food wrap and store in the refrigerator.

MORE SANDWICH SELECTIONS

- Lean ham, mustard, and lettuce.
- Lean beef, ½ tsp (2.5 ml) horseradish sauce, and greens.
- Chicken (white meat) and low-fat coleslaw (page 65).
- Lean ham, cottage cheese, and lettuce.
- Tuna fish, cucumber, green onions, and cilantro leaves.
- Low-fat feta cheese with sliced onion and lettuce.
- Goat cheese with watercress and tomato.
- Shrimp, avocado, and lemon juice.
- Chicken (white meat) in curried low-fat mayonnaise with chopped apple and light raisins.

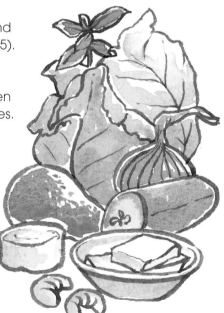

HELPFUL HEALTH TIPS

- Try to have fruit and a vitamin-packed drink, such as fresh fruit juice or fat-free milk, with your lunch to add to its nutritional value.

- See pages 60 and 61, for more quick-to-fix, but nutritional, lunchtime snacks.

- Instead of a sandwich, pack one of the salads on pages 65–66 in an airtight container.

- Soup is a good way to warm and fill up in the winter; make one of the Simple Soups, pages 68–69, and carry it in a vacuum flask.

- Use ground pepper, fresh herbs, spices, or mustard to pep up sandwiches. Choose whole wheat bread, which is higher in fiber and richer in vitamins and minerals.

- Supermarkets and delis usually carry low-fat, calorie-counted sandwiches. Choose fillings with plenty of lean meat, or fish, lettuce, or tomato. Avoid mayonnaise-based sandwiches.

Herbal Health

Be generous when adding herbs and spices to your food—they taste delicious, will not add calories, and are good for your health. As herbs and spices bring out the flavor of food, they are especially useful as a replacement for salt if you need to reduce your intake.

HERBS FOR FLAVOR

■ **Basil** Perfect in combination with tomato—make a low-fat, low-salt sauce by adding 2 tbsp basil (or basil and oregano) to a can of tomatoes, and simmering.

■ **Cilantro** Mix with boiled rice, throw into salads, add to stir-fries. Mix with tinned tuna (in spring water) for a low-fat sandwich or potato filling.

■ **Rosemary** Perfect with lamb (marinate with red wine and garlic). Add, with a little olive oil, to a tray of Mediterranean-style vegetables before roasting. Add a sprig to potatoes before baking.

■ **Tarragon** Coat chicken breasts with lemon juice, tarragon, and a dash of olive oil, wrap in aluminum foil, and cook; pour the same combination over vegetables or potatoes as a low-fat herb sauce.

■ **Dill** Complements fish and salads. Add to grated carrot together with a fat-free vinaigrette dressing. Make a tasty marinade for broiled fish by adding to lemon juice.

■ **Chamomile** Calm down with chamomile. This herb's mild sedative properties make it excellent for helping to reduce anxiety and aid sleep. Infuse a sachet of chamomile tea in freshly boiled water for 10–15 minutes to gain the full effects of the herb.

■ **Parsley** Help eliminate bad breath and PMS bloating with parsley. Parsley is a natural diuretic. Chewing on a sprig of fresh parsley also helps to subdue garlic-smelling breath by neutralizing odor-causing bacteria.

■ **Fennel** Fennel seeds, which taste a bit like licorice, help alleviate gas and have a calming effect on the gastrointestinal system. Simply chew ¼ tsp of these seeds, and swallow.

■ **Mint** Mint contains menthol, a digestive aid that can relieve gastrointestinal discomfort. Peppermint has antispasmodic properties that can help relieve bowel cramping. Make a cup of peppermint tea (available from most health food stores, supermarkets, and pharmacies) after a meal or put a few drops of peppermint extract in a glass of water and sip slowly.

■ **Garlic** and **chilies** Help fight a cold with garlic and chilies. Capsaicin in chilies is a decongestant and raw garlic has antiviral and antibacterial properties. Both may also be helpful in combating artery-clogging diseases. Adding a chopped chili and clove of garlic to a low-fat soup just before serving can help ease cold or flu symptoms.

■ Using herbs and spices in your food not only makes it taste better, it also means their flavors can replace that of salt. Salt is known to encourage water retention and hypertension or high blood pressure.

■ Ginger is an easily available and popular spice. It's well known for its zingy taste and anti-nausea benefits. Chew it raw, make ginger tea, add it to stir-fries and salads, and put it in the juicer with orange and carrot to make a great pick-me-up drink.

■ Dried herbs and spices are fine to use, but fresh ones do have a better flavor. If you can, create your own little herb garden so you always have your favorites to hand. You can freeze small-leaved herbs, such as rosemary and thyme. They do lose their texture, but retain much of their flavor. Chilies freeze particularly well. You can also buy freeze-dried fresh herbs, which are a good compromise.

Healthy Salads 1

Salads are a great way to boost your vitamin and mineral intake. This selection of salads is suitable for vegetarians, and the recipes are so tasty that they will soon be favorites with meat-eaters too.

CARROT & LEMON

You will need: *4 carrots, 3 tbsp currants, 2 green onions, 2 tbsp sunflower seeds, 1 tbsp/15 ml lemon juice, 1 tbsp/15 ml olive oil, 1 tsp/5 ml honey* **Serves 2**

1 Using the grater attachment on a food processor, grate the carrots. Mix in the currants and finely chopped green onions.
2 Whisk together the remaining ingredients with a little salt and freshly ground black pepper and toss into the carrots.

ORANGE & CHICORY

You will need: *2 heads chicory, 2 oranges, large handful watercress, 2 tbsp/30 ml store-bought, fat-free vinaigrette dressing* **Serves 2**

1 Separate and wash the chicory leaves and arrange on plates. Cut the peel and pith from the oranges and cut into chunks. Chop the watercress and mix with the oranges.
2 Pile the orange mixture over the chicory, add the salad dressing, and freshly ground black pepper.

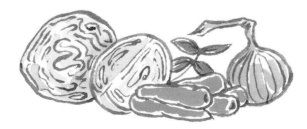

WARM MUSHROOM

You will need: *10 oz/300 g baby button mushrooms, 1 tbsp/15 ml soy sauce, 4 tbsp/60 ml water, 4 tbsp/60 ml tomato purée, 1 tbsp/15 ml white wine vinegar, 1 bay leaf, 1 garlic clove, 1 tbsp fresh chopped parsley* **Serves 2**

1 Wash the mushrooms and place in a large saucepan with the soy sauce, water, tomato purée, vinegar, bay leaf, and garlic. Bring to a boil and simmer for 5–7 minutes or until the mushrooms are tender and the sauce has thickened.
2 Stir in the parsley, and serve immediately or chill until required.

LOW-FAT COLESLAW

You will need: *¼ white cabbage, 2 carrots, 1 onion, 1 tbsp/15 ml fresh chopped tarragon, 2 tbsp/30 ml low-fat mayonnaise, 2 tbsp/30 ml low-fat yogurt* **Serves 2**

1 Shred the cabbage using the slicer attachment on a food processor, and grate the carrots and onion. Transfer to a bowl.
2 Mix the tarragon into the mayonnaise and low-fat yogurt; toss well into the salad.

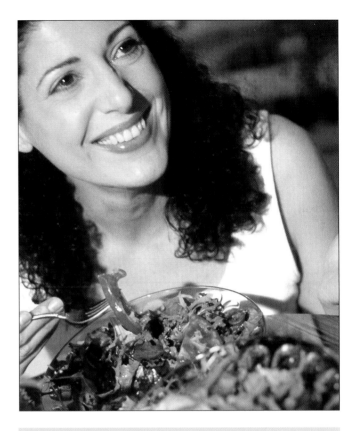

ZUCCHINI & BASIL

You will need: *3 zucchini, 1 orange, large handful washed baby leaf spinach, 2 tbsp fresh chopped basil, 2 tbsp/30 ml ready prepared fat-free garlic or vinaigrette dressing* **Serves 2**

1 Using the grater attachment on a food processor, coarsely grate the zucchini.
2 Cut the peel and pith from the orange and slice. Mix into the zucchini with the spinach and basil, and toss in the dressing.

HealthySalads2

Salads don't have to be just vegetables to be healthy—choose from chicken, fish, eggs, and low-fat cheese for healthy salads. The selection here ranges from the visually vibrant, Italian mozzarella and tomato salad to a substantial pasta salad with tuna.

MOZZARELLA & TOMATO

You will need: *10 oz/300 g low-fat mozzarella cheese, 2 large beef tomatoes, 4 tbsp/60 ml mixed pepper antipasto or canned pimiento, sliced, 1 tbsp basil leaves, 10 black olives, 1 tbsp/15 ml olive oil, sea salt* **Serves 2**

1 Slice the mozzarella and tomatoes and arrange on 2 plates. Scatter over the mixed pepper antipasto or pimiento, basil leaves, and olives.
2 Sprinkle over a little sea salt and plenty of freshly ground black pepper. Leave for 2 minutes, then drizzle over the olive oil.

SMOKED MACKEREL

You will need: *2 fillets smoked mackerel, 3 oz/90 g package mixed greens, 1 small raw beet, 2 green onions, chopped, 4 tsp/20 ml seasoned rice vinegar* **Serves 2**

1 Skin and flake the mackerel fillets. Place the mixed greens onto plates and top with the fish. Using the grater attachment on a blender, coarsely grate the beet and scatter over the top with the chopped green onions.
2 Drizzle a little seasoned rice vinegar over each serving.

HERBED WHEAT

You will need: *1 cup/4 oz/125 g bulgur wheat, large handful fresh parsley, large handful fresh mint, 4 green onions, ¼ cucumber, 1 tomato, 2 tbsp/30 ml lemon juice, 1 tbsp/15 ml olive oil* **Serves 2**

1 Pour 1 pint (300 ml) boiling water over the wheat, cover, and set aside for 8–10 minutes. Put the herbs and green onions into a food processor and blend until roughly chopped. Dice the cucumber.
2 Drain the wheat and rinse under cold water. Tip into a bowl and toss in the herbs, cucumber, lemon juice, chopped tomato, and oil. Add a little sea salt and plenty of freshly ground black pepper.

TUNA PASTA

You will need: *4 oz/125 g quick-cooking macaroni, 1 can (7 oz/200 g) tuna in spring water, 2 green onions, 2 tomatoes, 2 tbsp fresh chopped basil, 2 tbsp/30 ml low-fat mayonnaise, 2 tbsp/30 ml low-fat plain yogurt.* **Serves 2**

1 Cook the macaroni according to package directions, drain well, and rinse in cold water. Put in a bowl with the tuna, chopped green onion, chopped tomatoes, and basil.
2 Mix in the mayonnaise and yogurt, and season with plenty of freshly ground black pepper.

HELPFUL HEALTH TIPS

■ Buy a selection of greens; wash, and pack in food bags in the refrigerator. It is then easy to grab a handful at a moment's notice.

■ Add toasted poppy and sesame seeds to salads for a delicious flavor and nutty bite.

■ Avoid supermarket salad toppers such as bacon bits and croutons—they are full of hidden fat.

■ To make a salad more unusual, add blanched vegetables such as green beans and broccoli. They help to bulk it out and add valuable nutrients.

Low-fat Dressings

The salad dressing can triple the fat content of your meal if it is used to excess. To avoid piling on the calories, whisk up one of these light, low-fat dressings and keep it in a jar in the refrigerator for instant use. Completely fat-free vinaigrette dressing is best bought from the supermarket. For speed at home, drizzle rice wine or balsamic vinegar over your salad. Rice wine vinegar is light and not too acid; balsamic, although expensive, has a delicious flavor.

HONEYGAR VINAIGRETTE

You will need: ⅔ cup/5 fl oz/150 ml cider vinegar, 3 tbsp/ 45 ml honey, 4 tsp whole grain mustard, ½ cup/4 fl oz/125 ml light virgin olive oil, salt, black pepper
Makes 1¼ cups/10 fl oz/ 300 ml

1 Whisk everything together in a bowl with a little salt and plenty of freshly ground black pepper. Pour into a jar, seal, and keep in the refrigerator. Shake well before use.

YOGURT DRESSING

You will need: 1 cup/8 fl oz/250 ml low-fat yogurt, 2 tbsp/30 ml fat-free milk, 2 tbsp snipped chives, 1 garlic clove, grated rind of ½ lemon
Makes 1¼ cups/10 fl oz/300 ml

1 Blend together the low-fat yogurt and fat-free milk until smooth. Stir in the chives, garlic, and lemon rind. Add a little seasoning and store in the refrigerator.

CHEESE & CHIVES

You will need: 1¼ cups/10 fl oz/300 ml low-fat yogurt, 2 tbsp freshly grated Parmesan, 2 tbsp fresh chives, snipped, 1 tbsp chopped fresh parsley
Makes 1¼ cups/10 fl oz/ 300 ml

1 Whisk everything together in a bowl. Store in the refrigerator.

ORIENTAL DRESSING

You will need: ⅔ cup/5 fl oz/150 ml seasoned rice wine vinegar, 3 tbsp/45 ml clear honey, 2 tbsp/30 ml water, 2 tbsp/30 ml Thai fish sauce or light soy sauce, 2 green onions, finely chopped, 2 red and 2 green Thai chilies
Makes 1¼ cups/10 fl oz/300 ml

1 Heat the vinegar, honey, and water in a saucepan and boil for 1 minute. Stir in the fish or soy sauce, green onion, and thinly sliced chilies. Let cool, and store in the refrigerator.

LOW-CAL MAYONNAISE

You will need: 1 cup/8 fl oz/250 ml low-fat yogurt, 2 tsp German mustard, 1 tbsp/15 ml white wine vinegar, 4 tbsp/60 ml buttermilk ***Makes 1¼ cups/10 fl oz/300 ml***

1 Put the low-fat yogurt and mustard in a bowl with a little seasoning and gradually whisk in the vinegar and buttermilk until a mayonnaise consistency is achieved.

Variations:
- Stir in a little crushed garlic. Perfect to dip vegetables in.
- Chop some fresh mixed herbs and stir into the mixture.
- Add a dash of hot red pepper sauce and a little tomato paste. Excellent on shrimp.
- Stir in a little curry paste and toss into cooked chicken and chopped mango.

HELPFUL HEALTH TIPS

- Don't worry about using olive oil in dressings. Its benefits far outweigh its disadvantages. If you are on a low-calorie diet, don't use to excess.

- Look out for seasoned rice wine vinegar. It can be used as a dressing straight from the bottle.

- For 2 people use 1–2 tbsp/ 15–30 ml of dressing. You may need to add a little more creamy dressing to give a good coating but never more than 1 tablespoon of vinaigrette-style dressings.

- If using a strongly flavored dressing, you won't need much to lift a salad.

- Keep a selection of low-fat dressings in the refrigerator. You can also use them on hot pasta and rice dishes or as a sauce for broiled meats.

SimpleSoups1

It takes no time at all to make a bowl of soup and, though soups may look rich and filling, they are packed full of nutrients and can be a really healthy choice. Soup is a perfect way to start a meal as it will satisfy your initial hunger pangs, which in turn will help you to eat a smaller portion of the main course. Contrary to popular belief, soups don't need to be simmered for hours, provided you chop the ingredients finely at the start.

CREAMY MUSHROOM

You will need: 1 lb/450 g mixed mushrooms (flat, button, and chestnut), 1 cup/8 fl oz/250 ml dry sherry, 4 oz/125 g green onions, 2 garlic cloves, 2½ cups/1 pt/600 ml vegetable stock, 2 tbsp fresh chopped parsley, low-fat crème fraîche or low-fat sour cream to serve *Makes 5 cups/2 pt/1.2 liters*

1 Slice the mushrooms using the slicing blade on a food processor. Tip them into a large sauté pan with the sherry and cook over a high heat until the sherry has nearly evaporated.
2 Chop the green onions and garlic in the blender or food processor and add them to the mushrooms while they are cooking.
3 Add the broth and bring to a boil. Simmer for 5 minutes, stir in the parsley, and season to taste. Stir in a little crème fraîche or sour cream to serve.

PEA & LETTUCE

You will need: 1 tbsp/15 ml olive oil, 4 green onions, 8 oz/225 g frozen peas, 8 oz/225 g romaine lettuce, 1 tsp thyme leaves, 3¾ cups/1½ pt/850 ml boiling vegetable broth
Makes 5 cups/2 pt/1.2 liters

1 Heat the oil in a large saucepan and soften the green onion in it for 1 minute. Add the peas and cover with the broth. Bring to a boil and simmer for 3 minutes.
2 Finely shred the lettuce and stir into the soup with the thyme. Simmer 3 minutes more.
3 Blend until smooth and season to taste with ground black pepper.

CARROT & ORANGE

You will need: 1 tbsp/15 ml olive oil, 4 green onions, chopped, 1 tbsp ground cumin, 1 lb/500 g carrots, 3¾ cups/1½ pt/850 ml boiling vegetable broth, 1 orange *Makes 5 cups/2 pt/1.2 liters*

1 Using a large saucepan, cook the onions in the oil for 1 minute, then add the cumin. Peel and finely grate the carrots using the grater attachment on a food processor.
2 Add the carrots to the saucepan and cook over a high heat for 4 minutes. Add the broth and simmer for 5 minutes. Stir in the grated zest and juice from the orange and serve.

WATERCRESS

You will need: 1 leek, washed and thinly sliced, 1 large potato, peeled and finely diced, 5 oz/150 g watercress, 3¾ cups/1½ pt/850 ml boiling vegetable broth, freshly grated nutmeg
Makes 5 cups/2 pt/1.2 liters

1 Place the leek and potato in a large saucepan and pour over the broth. Bring to a boil and simmer for 8 minutes, or until the potato is just tender.
2 Stir in the watercress and bring back to a boil. Cover and simmer for 2 minutes. Pour into a blender and blend until smooth. Add a little nutmeg and seasoning to taste.

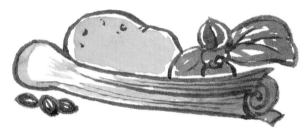

LEEK & POTATO

You will need: 1¼ lb/625 g leeks, 2 medium potatoes, 5 cups/2 pt/1.2 liters boiling vegetable broth *Makes 5 cups/2 pt/1.2 liters*

1 Thinly slice the leeks and wash well. Peel and finely dice the potatoes. Place them together in a pan with the boiling vegetable broth and simmer for 10 minutes.
2 Cool slightly, then blend in a food processor until smooth. Return to the pan, season to taste.

Simple Soups 2

The addition of herbs to a basic vegetable soup adds a wealth of flavor. These colorful soups all have a Mediterranean flavor and despite appearing quite luxurious, are simple and quick to prepare as well as being low in calories. Pack in a flask for a warming nutritious lunch at the office.

TOMATO & BASIL

You will need: *1 lb/500 g ripe sweet tomatoes, 1 sweet white onion, 2½ cups/1 pt/600 ml boiling vegetable broth, 3 tbsp fresh basil leaves, 1 tsp/5 ml honey, ⅔ cup/5 fl oz/150 ml low-fat crème fraîche or low-fat sour cream* **Makes 3¾ cups/1½ pt/850 ml**

1 Roughly chop the tomatoes and blend with the onion until smooth. Pour into a saucepan and add the boiling broth. Simmer for 10 minutes.
2 Stir in the basil, honey, and crème fraîche or sour cream. Season to taste.

VEGETABLE & BASIL

You will need: *15 oz/470 g shredded stir-fry vegetables, 3¾ cups/1½ pt/850 ml boiling vegetable broth, 2 tbsp/20 ml fresh basil leaves, 4 tbsp/60 ml freshly grated Parmesan cheese* **Makes 5 cups/2 pt/1.2 liters**

1 Put the vegetables and broth in a large saucepan and bring to a boil. Reduce the heat and simmer for 10 minutes.
2 Stir in the basil and season to taste. Scatter a little Parmesan cheese over each serving.

ZUCCHINI & MINT

You will need: *1 lb/500 g zucchini, 2 garlic cloves, 5 cups/2 pt/1.2 liters boiling vegetable broth, 2 tbsp freshly chopped mint, ⅔ cup/5 fl oz/150 ml low-fat yogurt* **Makes 5 cups/2 pt/1.2 liters**

1 Using the grater attachment on a food processor, grate the zucchini and tip into a saucepan. Add the crushed garlic and a splash of broth and cook, stirring often, until the zucchini soften.
2 Add the rest of the broth and bring to a boil. Simmer for 5 minutes. Add the mint and blend until smooth. Season to taste. Stir the yogurt into the warm soup and serve.

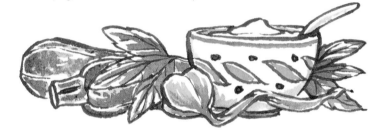

GAZPACHO

You will need: *1½ lb/750 g sweet ripe tomatoes, 3 slices bread, 2 tbsp/30 ml red wine vinegar, 3 garlic cloves, ½ cucumber, ½ sweet red pepper, 4 tbsp fresh chopped basil* **Makes 5 cups/2 pt/1.2 liters**

1 Place the tomatoes, bread, vinegar, and garlic in a food processor and blend until smooth. Gradually add 1¼ cups/10 fl oz/300 ml cold water until it forms a creamy consistency.
2 Add the cucumber and pepper to the blender and blend briefly. Stir in the basil and season to taste.

HELPFUL HEALTH TIPS

■ Don't be afraid to splash in a little alcohol for extra flavor as the cooking process will burn off those alcohol calories, leaving your soup with a special flavor.

■ Freeze soup in single portions so you always have some on hand even if you only need one serving.

■ Always use potato for thickening if needed. It adds body and nutrients at the same time.

■ If you like creamy soups, use low-fat yogurt, or low-fat versions of crème fraîche, or sour cream as substitutes for heavy cream.

■ If you prefer a chunky, hearty soup, you can purée half the soup and stir it into the rest.

FastSauces1

The joy of basic pasta sauces is that they are speedy, nutritious, and don't have to be served on pasta to be enjoyed. Any of them can also be spooned over baked potatoes, stirred into cooked rice, or served on bulgur wheat. The rules are simple. Reduce the amount of fat when frying anything—a teaspoon of oil at the most, if you use a non-stick skillet. If you have a craving for a creamy sauce, use low-fat yogurt, fromage frais or low-fat sour cream in place of heavy cream.

TOMATO & SPINACH CHILI

You will need: 1 garlic clove, minced, 1 tsp/5 ml olive oil, 8 halves sun-dried tomatoes, diced, 1 can (14 oz/400 g) chopped tomatoes, 3 oz/90 g fresh baby leaf spinach, 10 black olives, dash hot red pepper sauce **Serves 2**

1 Cook the garlic briefly in the olive oil. Pour boiling water over the sun-dried tomatoes and leave to soak for 5 minutes.
2 Add the chopped tomatoes to the garlic and cook for 5 minutes.
3 Add the spinach and drained and chopped sun-dried tomatoes to the sauce and boil rapidly for 5 minutes. Add the olives and a couple of dashes of hot red pepper sauce. Season to taste with salt and freshly ground black pepper.

BROCCOLI & SALMON

You will need: 5 oz/150 g tiny broccoli florets, 2 green onions, chopped, ⅔ cup/5 fl oz/150 ml fat-free milk, 1½ tsp cornstarch, ⅔ cup/5 fl oz/150 ml low-fat plain yogurt, 1 can (7 oz/200 g) red salmon, drained, squeeze lemon juice, 1 tsp dried dill **Serves 2**

1 Blanch the broccoli in boiling water for 4 minutes. Put the green onions and milk in a saucepan and bring to the boil. Blend the cornstarch with a little cold milk and stir into the saucepan until thickened.
2 Add the blanched broccoli florets and the remaining ingredients, and season to taste.

TUNA & ARTICHOKE

You will need: 2 garlic cloves, minced, ⅔ cup/5 fl oz/150 ml tomato purée, 6 canned artichoke halves, sliced, 1 can (4¼ oz/120 g) tuna in water, 1 tbsp drained capers, 1 tbsp fresh chopped basil **Serves 2**

1 Put the garlic and tomato purée in a saucepan and heat together for 2 minutes. Add the artichokes, flaked tuna, and capers, and bring to a boil. Stir in the basil and season to taste.

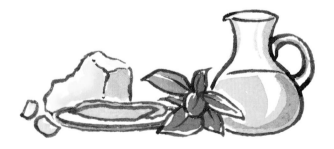

SMOKED HAM & BASIL

You will need: 2 garlic cloves, minced, 1 tsp/5 ml olive oil, 5 fl oz/150 ml low-fat yogurt, 2 tbsp/30 ml fat-free milk, 3 oz/90 g wafer-thin smoked ham, 2 tbsp Parmesan cheese, 1 tbsp fresh basil **Serves 2**

1 Cook the garlic briefly in the oil. Add the yogurt, milk, chopped ham, and grated cheese. Heat gently until just warm, then add the basil and season to taste.

MIXED SEAFOOD & DILL

You will need: grated rind of ½ lemon, 6 tbsp/90 ml white wine, 5 oz/150 g mixed seafood, 6 tbsp/90 ml fromage frais or low-fat yogurt, 1 tsp dried dill **Serves 2**

1 Put the lemon rind and white wine in a saucepan and bring to a boil. Simmer until reduced by half, then stir in the mixed seafood.
2 Heat through briefly, then stir in the fromage frais or low-fat yogurt and dill. Season to taste.

MEDITERRANEAN VEGETABLE

You will need: 1 small onion, chopped, 2 garlic cloves, minced, 1 zucchini, sliced, 1 tsp/5 ml olive oil, 1 can (7 oz/200 g) chopped tomatoes, 3½ oz/100 g drained canned chick peas, 1 tsp chopped fresh rosemary **Serves 2**

1 Cook the onion, garlic, and zucchini in the oil for 5 minutes. Add the tomatoes, chick peas, and rosemary, and bring to a boil. Simmer for 5 minutes, then season to taste with salt and freshly ground black pepper.

Fast Sauces 2

These basic sauces are good enough to serve just as they are, with pasta or rice, but for a change, try the variations suggested, stir different flavors of your choice into them at the last minute, or use them as a base from which to make other dishes.

NEAPOLITAN TOMATO

You will need: *2 onions, 2 garlic cloves, ½ tsp/2.5 ml paprika, ⅖ cup/5 fl oz/50 ml red wine, ½ tsp each dried thyme and oregano, 2 cans (14 oz/400 g) chopped tomatoes, 1 tbsp chopped parsley, 1 tbsp/15 ml tomato paste* **Serves 4**

1 Blend the onion and garlic together in a food processor. Scrape into a large saucepan and add the paprika and red wine. Bring to a boil and cook rapidly until nearly all the liquid has reduced and the onions are tender.
2 Add the thyme, oregano, and tomatoes, and bring to a boil. Simmer for 10 minutes, then stir in the parsley and tomato paste and season to taste.

Variations:
- *Spread thinly onto pita rounds, top with slices of low-fat mozzarella, and cook under the broiler until golden. Scatter over a few fresh basil leaves before serving.*
- *Blanch some mixed vegetables and stir into the sauce with canned lentils.*
- *Serve in baked or microwaved potatoes topped with a sprinkling of Parmesan cheese.*

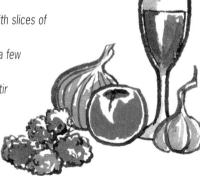

TURKEY BOLOGNESE

You will need: *1 lb/500 g turkey, ground, 1 carrot, ⅖ cup/ 5 fl oz/150 ml red wine, 1 jar (10 oz/290 g) mixed pepper antipasto or canned pimiento, sliced, 1 can (14 oz/400 g) chopped tomatoes, 1 tsp/5 ml dried mixed herbs, 2 tbsp/30 ml tomato paste* **Serves 4**

1 Heat a large sauté pan and add the turkey. Cook over a high heat until the turkey has browned. Grate the carrot and add to the turkey in the pan. Cook for 2 minutes.
2 Add the red wine, antipasto or pimiento, chopped tomatoes, herbs, and tomato paste. Bring to a boil and simmer for 10 minutes. Season to taste.

Variations:
- *Layer with cooked lasagne and top with slices of tomatoes and low-fat mozzarella. Bake in the oven or microwave until golden and bubbling.*
- *Spoon onto steamed bulgur wheat, with lemon juice, sunflower seeds, and parsley.*
- *Serve on baked or microwaved potatoes with a large fresh side salad.*

LOW-FAT PESTO

You will need: *3 oz/90 g fresh basil leaves, 1 oz/30 g fresh parsley, 4 tbsp freshly grated Parmesan, 1 oz/30 g toasted pine nuts, 4 garlic cloves, 8 oz/250 g quark, or reduced fat soft cheese, ⅖ cup/5 fl oz/150 ml low-fat yogurt* **Serves 4**

1 Put all the ingredients into a food processor and blend until smooth. Season to taste. Scrape into a container and keep in the refrigerator for up to 1 week.

Variations:
- *Spread onto toast and top with smoked salmon and a grinding of fresh black pepper.*
- *Soften mixed mushrooms in a pan with a little stock. Stir in some pesto and serve on baked or microwaved potatoes.*

HELPFUL HEALTH TIPS

- Toss one of these sauces into hot pasta, then leave to cool. Pack up as a tasty pasta salad for lunch.

- Prepare the make-ahead sauces in bulk and freeze in individual portions. This makes them perfect to thaw in the microwave and jazz up at a moment's notice.

- Choose fast-cooking fresh pasta that will be ready in the time it takes to make the sauce.

- Look out for filled pastas with low-fat fillings such as fat-free ricotta and spinach, or mushroom and garlic. In general, the vegetarian varieties will be lower in fat but cheese-filled pasta is the exception to the rule. Check the package for the nutritional table showing fat content per portion.

Ten-minute Dinners 1

When you have worked late and are ready to pick up a take-out for dinner, think again and whip up a nutritional meal instead. It can be done with very little effort and you'll feel better afterward. Stir-fries, vegetable bakes, pastas, baked potatoes cooked in the microwave, and broiled meats and fish can all be low in fat and are simple to cook.

SPEEDY STIR-FRY

You will need: *6 oz/175 g skinless chicken breast, cut into thin strips, 2 garlic cloves, minced, 1 tsp/5 ml olive oil, 10 oz/ 300 g frozen stir-fry vegetables, 1 tbsp peanut butter, 1 tbsp/15 ml dark soy sauce, ½ tsp minced chili* **Serves 2**

1 Heat a wok or large skillet and stir-fry the chicken and garlic in the oil for 2 minutes. Add the shredded vegetables and continue to cook over a high heat for 5 minutes or until just tender.
2 Blend the remaining ingredients together with 2 tbsp (30 ml) hot water and add to the pan. Cover and simmer for 1 minute.

PEPPERED PORK FILLET

You will need: *8 oz/250 g pork tenderloin, black pepper, 4 oz/125 g button mushrooms, 1 stalk celery, finely sliced, 2 green onions, finely chopped, 4 tbsp/60 ml dry white wine, 4 tbsp/60 ml low-fat crème fraîche or low-fat sour cream* **Serves 2**

1 Coat the pork with black pepper and a little salt. Cut into ½-in (1-cm) slices. Heat a heavy non-stick skillet and cook the pork over a high heat for 3 minutes turning once. Remove from the pan and set aside.
2 Add the mushrooms and celery to the skillet. Cook for 2 minutes until starting to soften. Add the onions and wine, simmer for 2 minutes. Stir in the crème fraîche or sour cream. Heat through and serve with the pork.

FIVE-SPICE STEAKS

You will need: *2 4-oz/125-g quick-fry steaks, 1 tsp 5-spice powder, 1 tsp/5 ml sesame oil, 10 oz/300 g frozen stir-fry vegetables, 1 tbsp/15 ml light soy sauce* **Serves 2**

1 Coat the steaks on both sides with 5-spice powder and plenty of ground black pepper. Heat the sesame oil in a large non-stick skillet and cook the vegetables for 5 minutes over a high heat until tender.
3 Divide between dinner plates, then return the pan to the heat. Add the steaks and cook over a high heat for 1–2 minutes on each side. Put a steak on each pile of vegetables and drizzle over a little soy sauce.

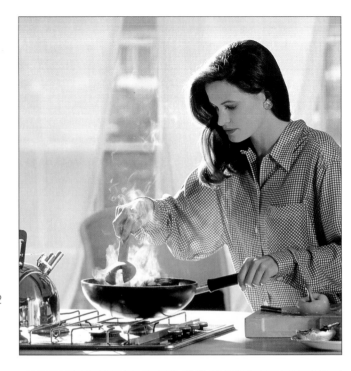

SPICY POTATO CURRY

You will need: *1 onion, finely sliced, 8 oz/250 g precooked sliced potatoes, 1 tsp/5 ml sunflower oil, 1 garlic clove, minced, 1 can (13 oz/400 g) chick peas, 1 tbsp tikka or curry paste, juice of ½ lemon, ⅔ cup/5 fl oz/150 ml boiling vegetable broth, ⅔ cup/5 fl oz/150 ml low-fat yogurt, 2 tbsp chopped fresh cilantro* **Serves 2**

1 Soften the onion and potatoes in the oil for 3 minutes. Add the garlic, chick peas, and tikka or curry paste, and cook, stirring often, for 3 minutes.
2 Add the lemon juice and broth, cover and simmer for 10 minutes. Stir in the yogurt and cilantro.

Ten-minute Dinners 2

Fish, seafood, and vegetables combine to make these recipes delicious, nutritious and fast to prepare. When you can make a meal in minutes, there's no reason to buy takeout meals.

SMOKED HADDOCK FLORENTINE

You will need: *2 5-oz/150-g smoked haddock fillets, fat-free milk, 7 oz/215 g leaf spinach, pinch grated nutmeg, 2 tomatoes, 3½ oz/100 g low-fat mozzarella* **Serves 2**

1 Put the haddock in enough milk just to cover and bring to a boil. Simmer for 2 minutes, then drain, and place the fillets in a braising dish. Cook the spinach, with just a little nutmeg, in a large saucepan until wilted, then squeeze out all the liquid.
2 Top each fish fillet with spinach and a layer of sliced tomatoes. Finish with a layer of mozzarella and broil until golden and bubbling.

SEAFOOD RISOTTO

You will need: *2 tbsp/30 ml dry white wine, 4 tbsp/60 ml boiling vegetable broth, 1 package (14 oz/430 g) frozen rice with vegetables, 6 oz/175 g mixed seafood, ½ tsp dried dill* **Serves 2**

1 Bring the broth and wine to a boil in a large sauté pan, add the rice, and simmer for 5 minutes.
2 Add the seafood and dill. Cover and continue to cook for 3 minutes, or until the rice is tender and all the broth has been absorbed.

SHREDDED VEGETABLE PILAF

You will need: *1 tbsp/15 ml olive oil, 10 oz/300 g mixed vegetables, shredded, 2 tbsp pumpkin seeds, 8 oz/250 g cooked rice, ⅔ cup/5 fl oz/150 ml boiling vegetable broth, 8 dried apricots, chopped, 1 tbsp chopped fresh parsley* **Serves 2**

1 Heat the oil in a large sauté pan. Add the vegetables and pumpkin seeds. Stir over a high heat for 2–3 minutes.
2 Add the rice, broth, and apricots and cook for 3–4 minutes or until all the broth has been absorbed and the rice is tender. Stir in the parsley and season to taste.

SHRIMP, GARLIC & CHILI

You will need: *8 oz/250 g large shelled and deveined shrimp, 3 garlic cloves, sliced, 1 Thai red chili, sliced, 1 tsp/5 ml olive oil, ½ lemon, 2 large handfuls mixed salad leaves, 1 avocado, sliced, chopped parsley to garnish (optional)* **Serves 2**

1 Cook the shrimp, garlic, and chili in the oil for 2 minutes. Do not let the garlic burn or it will taste bitter. Squeeze over the lemon juice and season to taste.
2 Divide the salad leaves and avocado between 2 plates and top with the shrimp and some parsley.

HELPFUL HEALTH TIPS

■ Purchase meats prepared for cooking, such as ground turkey, stir-fry chicken strips, lean pork, and quick-fry beef steaks.

■ Use a heavy-based, non-stick skillet and you'll be surprised how little, if any, fat needs to be added.

■ Reduce the amount of meat in a meal and make up the weight with vegetables.

■ Brown meats without any fat. If the meat starts to stick, add a little broth rather than oil.

■ Fresh fish is the ultimate healthy fast food. Squeeze a little citrus juice over, cover with aluminum foil and bake in a hot oven.

■ A meal doesn't have to be focused on meat or fish. Serve vegetable recipes with crusty whole wheat bread.

Ten-minute Desserts 1

You can eat healthily and still indulge in delicious desserts. If you like to finish the meal with something sweet, there are many ways to satisfy that craving without resorting to sugary desserts full of empty calories. If you want to be a bit more adventurous without spending hours in the kitchen, these fruit-based desserts provide vitamins, minerals, and a luxurious taste that is suitable for entertaining.

BAKED BANANAS

You will need: *2 large bananas, 2 tbsp/30 ml maple syrup, 4 pecan halves, chopped, pinch ground cinnamon* **Serves 2**

1 Peel and thickly slice the bananas. Place in a flameproof dish and sprinkle over the maple syrup, chopped pecan nuts, and a pinch of ground cinnamon.
2 Place the dish under a hot broiler for 2 minutes. Serve with low-fat yogurt.

FRUITY MERINGUES

You will need: *⅔ cup/5 fl oz/150 ml low-fat yogurt, 1 tbsp/15 ml honey, 2 meringue nests, 4 oz/125 g mixed summer berries (such as strawberries, blueberries, and raspberries), 1 tsp confectioners' sugar* **Serves 2**

1 Mix the yogurt and honey together and spoon into the meringue nests.
2 Top with a selection of the berries and dust with a little confectioners' sugar just before serving.

BROILED PEACHES

You will need: *2 peaches, 1 tbsp/15 ml honey, 3 tbsp/45 ml ricotta cheese, 2 amaretti cookies, crumbled* **Serves 2**

1 Halve and remove pit from the peaches, and place them in a small flameproof dish. Drizzle over the honey and put under a hot broiler for 2 minutes.
2 Mix the ricotta cheese and amaretti cookies and spoon into the centers of the peaches. Return to the broiler and cook until lightly golden.

BLUEBERRY BRULÉE

You will need: *4 oz/125 g blueberries, 4 tbsp/60 ml low-fat yogurt, and 4 tbsp/60 ml fromage frais, or 8 tbsp/120 ml low-fat yogurt, ½ tsp/2.5 ml vanilla extract, 4 tsp soft dark brown sugar* **Serves 2**

1 Put the blueberries in the bottom of 2 ramekin dishes. Mix the yogurt, fromage frais, and vanilla extract, and spoon onto the fruit.
2 Scatter the sugar over the top of each and cook under a hot broiler until the sugar has melted.

SPICED PLUMS & PINEAPPLE

You will need: *3 eating plums, sliced, 6 oz /150 g fresh prepared pineapple, pinch grated nutmeg, 6 tbsp/90 ml low-fat crème fraîche or low-fat sour cream, 2 tbsp soft light brown sugar* **Serves 2**

1 Mix the fruits together and spoon onto 2 dessert plates. Sprinkle over some nutmeg and spoon the crème fraîche or sour cream on top.
2 Sprinkle the sugar over each serving and let stand for 10 minutes before eating.

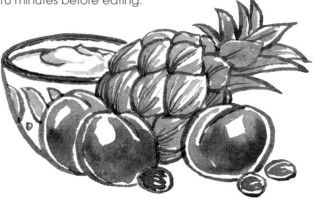

GINGER MELON MEDLEY

You will need: *½ cantaloupe melon, ½ charentais melon, ¼ watermelon, 2 pieces stem ginger* **Serves 2**

1 Cut the peel from the melons and scoop out the seeds. Cut the fruit into chunky pieces and divide between 2 bowls.
2 Cut the ginger into fine dice and scatter over the top of the melons.

Ten-minute Desserts2

Enjoy fruits in season, or for an occasional treat look for exotic fruit ingredients, such as pawpaw, passion fruit, and mango.

POACHED PEARS

You will need: *1½ cups/12 fl oz/350 ml red grape juice, ½ tsp/2.5 ml vanilla extract, 2 tbsp/30 ml honey, grated zest of 1 orange, 1 cinnamon stick, 2 pears* **Serves 2**

1 Combine the grape juice, vanilla, honey, orange zest, and cinnamon. Bring to a boil and simmer for 5 minutes.
2 Peel and core the pears and cut into thick wedges. Add to the grape juice, cover, and simmer for 5 minutes. Serve warm, or let cool and keep in the refrigerator until required.

CHERRIES IN HONEYED YOGURT

You will need: *1 can (14 oz/400 g) black cherries, grated rind of ½ orange, 1 carton (7 fl oz/200 ml) fromage frais or low-fat yogurt, 1 tbsp/15 ml clear honey, a few drops almond extract, 2 tsp light brown sugar* **Serves 2**

1 Drain and rinse the cherries, divide between 2 small braising dishes. Top with a little orange zest.
2 Mix the fromage frais or low-fat yogurt, honey, and almond extract and spoon over the cherries. Top with a little sugar.

LOW-FAT LEMON SYLLABUB

You will need: *2 tbsp/30 ml white wine, 1 tbsp/15 ml lemon cordial, ½ lime, grated zest only, 1⅓ cups/ 10 fl oz/300 ml low-fat yogurt* **Serves 2**

1 Mix the white wine and lemon cordial in a large bowl with the lime zest.
2 Gradually whisk the yogurt into the wine mixture. Serve with reduced-fat dessert cookies.

EXOTIC FRUIT KEBABS

You will need: *1 small mango, peeled, 1 small pawpaw, peeled and deseeded, 4 oz/125 g ready-prepared fresh pineapple, pinch ground cinnamon, 1 tbsp light brown sugar, 1 passion fruit* **Serves 2**

1 Cut the mango flesh from the pit and then into large chunks, and cut the pawpaw into similar-size pieces. Thread alternately with the pineapple onto 4 wooden skewers.
2 Place the skewers on a broiler rack and sprinkle over the cinnamon and sugar. Cook under a hot broiler until they start to color.
3 Meanwhile, press the passion fruit seeds through a sieve to release their juice. Pour over the fruit before serving.

TIPS

■ You will find a wide range of low-fat yogurts, ice creams, frozen yogurts, and sorbets in supermarkets. It's vital to check the fat and sugar content on the package. Some products may be labeled low-fat but can still contain an incredible amount of sugar.

■ When you are eating out, the best option is always a fruit salad, but resist the urge to cover it with cream.

■ If you are on a reduced-calorie diet, it is important to reduce the sugar as well as the fat content of your diet. It is much better to opt for desserts that have natural sweetness such as poached pears and mixed fruit medleys.

■ Make sure desserts have nutritional value as well as being good to eat. You can then end a meal with a satisfied glow.

Eat, Drink & Relax To Sleep

One of the most common complaints of our time is tiredness and problems with sleeping. There are many reasons for sleep being disrupted, including stress, alcohol, some prescription or recreational drugs, nicotine, external noise, going to bed hungry, going to bed too full, illness, pain, and so on, but there are certain foods, drinks and techniques that may help you to sleep better than others.

TEN WAYS TO EAT AND SLEEP WELL

1 Eat regularly
Eating regular meals at regular times can be more important than eating or drinking specific things before bed, so try to get into a routine.

2 Cut the caffeine
Caffeine is one of the major causes of insomnia. Try to cut down on tea, coffee, and cola consumption during the day and avoid them altogether in the evenings, especially strong cups of tea or coffee.

3 Less liquid
Try not to consume too much liquid shortly before going to bed to avoid being awakened by the need to go to the bathroom. Before bed, make a relaxing herbal tea, or one containing ginseng, in a small teacup.

4 Avoid too much alcohol
A glass of wine with your meal, or the occasional alcoholic nightcap, should not do you any harm if you normally sleep well. Avoid too much alcohol, however, as it will interfere with the quality of your sleep.

5 Serotonin for sleep
A small snack containing carbohydrate, calcium, and magnesium, such as a cracker, a banana, and some yogurt, is thought to be the best bedtime snack. These foods help to produce serotonin in your brain, which is key for sleep. Some studies have claimed that an amino acid called tryptophan can help to beat insomnia and improve sleep. It is difficult, however, to take tryptophan in sufficient quantities through food alone, so it is most often taken as a supplement.

6 Essential calming aromas
Essential oils can induce sleep—see Calming Scents page 88.

7 Learn to relax
The techniques used in Think Tranquility, page 86, Meditation for Calm, page 90, Deep Breathing, page 94, and Essential Daily Relaxation, page 98, are all highly effective in inducing sleep.

8 Exercise to sleep
Exercising in the late afternoon or early evening can help you sleep more soundly. Don't exercise less than 2 to 3 hours before bed.

9 Deal with stress
Anxiety and stress are among the most common reasons for insomnia and disrupted sleep. Try to deal with your stress before going to bed. Use some of the relaxing exercises in Section 4—Calm & Relax.

10 Don't just lie there
If you don't fall asleep within 20 minutes, get up and watch television or read a book.

Foods to Help You Snooze

AVOID BEFORE BED
- Alcohol
- Nicotine
- Caffeine
- A heavy meal, especially spicy or fatty food
- High-protein foods, such as red meat or cheese

TRY BEFORE BED
- A small carbohydrate snack
- Herbal drinks and teas. Choose from chamomile, valerian, peppermint or orange bergamot tea, or one containing ginseng

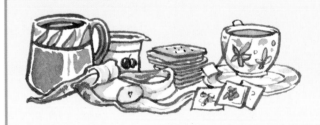

Eat Vegetarian

Following a vegetarian diet, or reducing the amount of meat you eat, can improve your health. A well-balanced vegetarian diet, like any other, should be low in fat, and high in fiber, carbohydrates, vitamins and minerals.

VEGETARIAN FACTS

1 What is a vegetarian?
There are different types of vegetarian. One group, often called vegetarians, are more correctly called lacto-ovo-vegetarians. They eat vegetables, fruit, nuts, dairy products, and eggs. They do not eat meat, fish or seafood. Lacto-vegetarians also cut eggs from their diet. Vegans (strict vegetarians) eat no animal products at all.

2 A healthy option
Keeping meat-free helps protect against a range of problems, including cancer, coronary artery disease, high blood pressure, and diabetes, as well as making you less likely to become obese.

3 A balanced diet
A well-balanced vegetarian diet is based on three main food groups: grains, beans, seeds, nuts, and tofu; leafy green vegetables; and other vegetables and fruits.

4 Healthier than a meat-eater?
As with any healthy diet, avoid dishes that are fried, breaded, covered in heavy cream, or loaded with salt. Avoid salad dressings not fat free or low fat.

5 The protein problem
A combination of grains and legumes provide protein, as do eggs and dairy products, such as milk and cheese. Many people eat twice as much animal protein as they need. Experts in nutrition warn that such high meat and animal fat consumption has resulted in the increasing rates of heart disease, stroke, and cancer.

6 Getting enough iron?
There is some controversy over whether vegetarians are at risk from anemia because they lack essential iron in their diet. (Red meat is one of the richest and most easily absorbed sources of iron.) You can get iron from many vegetarian sources, including leafy green vegetables, dried fruits, soybeans, whole grains, and molasses. You can significantly increase your iron intake by cooking in iron pots. Also, if you eat or drink vitamin C-rich foods (tomatoes, orange juice, green vegetables) with an iron-rich food you can greatly increase iron absorption.

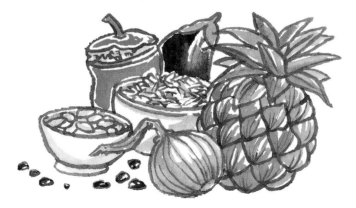

7 Vitamins and minerals
A vegetarian diet may be low in vitamin B12, vitamin D, calcium, and zinc. So, eat a well-balanced diet and :
- Drink calcium-fortified soy milk or fat-free cow's milk.
- Eat a wide variety of foods from each of the food groups.
- Follow the guidelines outlined on page 52.
- Choose an iron-fortified breakfast cereal.
- Take a vitamin B12 supplement.

8 Tasty and nutritious
The variety of fresh vegetables, fruit, and nuts available means that a vegetarian diet need never be boring. Experiment with "exotic" vegetables, such as celeriac, a celery-flavored root vegetable, fennel with its mild aniseed flavor, or okra, delicious in stir-fries or curries.

9 Meat-free meat
If you love the taste and texture of meat, experiment with some of the meat substitutes available at health food stores, such as tofu or texturized protein products.

10 Vegetarian family
A balanced vegetarian diet is suitable for all the family. However, you should consult a doctor and a registered dietitian before putting a child on a vegan diet. Vegans should also plan for pregnancy by modifying their diets and taking supplements as advised by an obstetrician.

HealthBoosters

Healthy eating really can help protect you against serious diseases such as heart disease and cancers. A well-balanced diet, high in calcium and magnesium, can also help maintain strong bones and guard against osteoporosis, while other nutrients have been shown to minimize the effects of PMS.

MINIMIZE PMS

■ Premenstrual syndrome, or PMS, is the name for the symptoms that occur just before your monthly period. Diet can help ease the irritability, breast tenderness, headaches, tiredness, bloating, sugar cravings, and mood swings that often accompany the monthly cycle.

■ Eat plenty of complex carbohydrate foods, fresh fruits, and vegetables to make sure you are getting essential minerals and vitamins (especially iron, lost during menstruation, and B-complex vitamins). Try to beat your cravings for chocolates and cakes. Replace these foods with more nutritious sweet flavors, such as dried apricots and bananas. Preventing swings in your blood-sugar levels should help to even out your moods.

■ Cut down on animal fats and salt since they're directly related to water retention, which can make premenstrual bloating worse. Cut down on caffeine, processed foods, and alcohol too.

STRONG BONES

■ Until quite recently people assumed that shrunken, brittle bones were a natural sign of aging. The latest research shows that this is not the case. Many more women in their fifties and sixties are suffering prematurely from the bone disease osteoporosis. The disease occurs when bones lose the calcium they need to keep them strong. Bones become thin, porous, and brittle, causing pain, deformity and fractures.

■ The key to preventing osteoporosis is a constant supply of calcium—particularly during childhood. Calcium can be found in many foods, including leafy green vegetables, beans, nuts, dairy products, and canned fish with softened bones. All milk is high in calcium, but fat-free and low-fat milk have the same amount of calcium as whole milk but less of the saturated fat. If you feel you are not getting enough calcium in your diet, consult your doctor about taking a supplement.

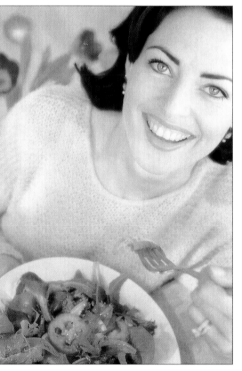

■ Exercising throughout your life helps the calcium to strengthen and build bones.

■ Cut down on caffeine, alcohol, and smoking as they may speed the loss of calcium from the body.

SUPER VITAMINS

■ Antioxidant vitamins (A, derived from betacarotene, C, and E) mop up free radicals in your body that can damage tissues and cells, causing diseases, such as heart disease and certain cancers, as well as signs of aging. Enriching your diet with foods high in these vitamins will help you and your family stay healthy. Maximize your daily intake by following these guidelines.

■ Betacarotene is the precursor to Vitamin A. It is found in most fruits and vegetables with an orange-yellow pigment. Carrots, sweet yellow peppers, sweet potatoes, pumpkin, cantaloupes, and apricots are good sources of betacarotene.

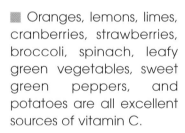

■ Oranges, lemons, limes, cranberries, strawberries, broccoli, spinach, leafy green vegetables, sweet green peppers, and potatoes are all excellent sources of vitamin C.

■ Include plenty of wheat germ, sunflower seeds, whole grain cereals, whole wheat bread, and safflower oil in your diet to get all the vitamin E you need to stay healthy.

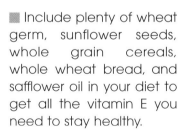

4 Calm&Relax

Beat Stress **Take It Easy**

Taking just 10 minutes a day to unwind will help to make both your mind and body healthier. It will make you feel happier, too! If you don't relax, stress can start to affect your health—headaches, depression, insomnia, poor concentration, irritability, indigestion, skin problems, and constant tiredness are all symptoms of stress.

Try this simple stress test as you are reading this page. Can you drop your shoulders down? Are you frowning? Are your teeth clenched or your lips pursed? Are any of your muscles tight and tense?

If you answered "yes" to any of these questions, or frequently get stomach upsets, headaches, backache, or suffer from general muscular aches and pains, you probably need to improve your stress-relieving strategies.

Many of the physical and mental stresses we suffer are caused by a fast-paced but

COPING sedentary lifestyle. If you spend the day sitting hunched over a keyboard or telephone and then sit in a car, driving home in heavy traffic, you are bound to feel tired and tense. You probably just want to relax with your feet up watching a movie or television program, or out at a bar with friends—but try to find 10 minutes to follow a simple relaxation routine first. It will make you feel calmer and fresher and be much better for your long-term health.

Exercise is the simplest and most effective antidote to stress. Without exercise, our muscles become stiff and tense and our breathing shallow. If you usually spend most

BREATHE of the day sitting down and don't get much exercise, turn to the pages illustrating stretches and deep breathing techniques. If you have been rushing from place to place and need to calm down, check out the meditation and visualization ideas, or work through the essential daily

UNWIND relaxer to unwind your whole body.

In this section you will also find many strategies for relaxing different parts of your body. Many of these exercises and techniques can be done during the day, even while you are at work or traveling. Find your favorites and use them regularly.

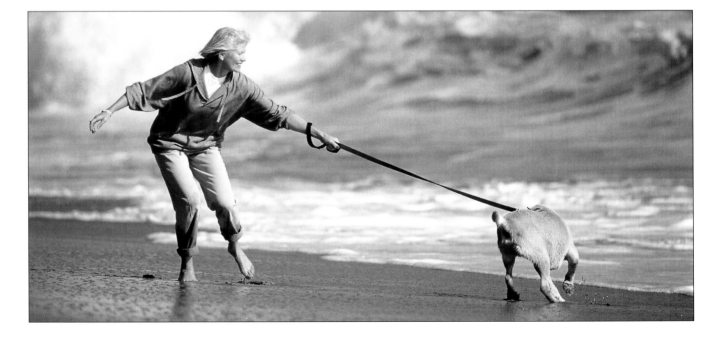

StressproofYourLife

Everyone knows that stress damages your health. It causes a range of physical symptoms, from aching muscles, headaches, and eczema to potentially fatal heart disease and strokes. Stress affects appearance, too—it makes spots flare up, skin dry and gray-tinged, and causes dark rings under the eyes. When you're tense, you frown and clench your teeth, too—neither are beauty enhancers! Here are some simple ideas for leading a stress-free life.

TOP TEN ANTI-STRESS TECHNIQUES

1 Remain physically and mentally active
Take some form of exercise every day. A 10-minute walk or a few minutes' running on the spot will make a difference. Read a newspaper or listen to news reports. Do crosswords or other puzzles when you are on a journey or waiting in line.

2 Plan and prioritize
When you feel overwhelmed by everything you have to do, make a list. Prioritize the essentials, ignore the inessentials, and longterm, make an effort to delegate some of your chores—whether it's housework or office work.

3 Be realistic
Many of us take on too much—learn to say no.

4 Take short breaks
Short rest periods, just five or 10 minutes throughout the day, will refresh your mind and body. Try to get outdoors. If that isn't possible, walk around the house or office, or do a few stretches at your desk.

5 Treat yourself
Take the telephone off the hook and relax in a candlelit bath. Buy yourself flowers, or a small treat such as an aromatherapy candle.

6 Don't brood
Going over past mistakes and worrying about the future can internalize stress. Give yourself permission, for just one day, not to think about the past or worry about the future. You will enjoy yourself so much it should become a habit! If you find yourself slipping into worry mode, work through your favorite relaxation technique.

7 Keep a sense of humor
Laughter is one of the best antidotes to stress. Keep a collection of books, articles, videos, funny family photographs—anything that makes you smile. Look at them when you feel down. Remember which friends make you laugh and treat yourself to an evening with positive people!

8 Accentuate the positive
Make an effort to take a more positive approach to life. If you feel overwhelmed by

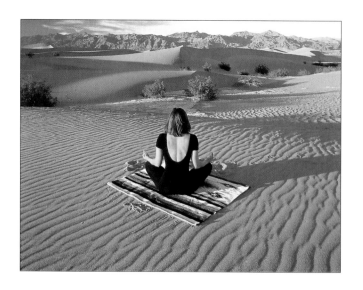

negative thoughts, find 10 minutes to do some of the exercises in Section 1—Get Moving! or try one of the positive visualizations on pages 86 and 87—even a few minutes can help to lighten your mood and give you the incentive to do an energizing exercise routine.

9 Talk about problems
Don't store anger and let it. build up into resentment. Work out your pent-up aggression—run up and down the stairs or visualize your angry thoughts blowing away as you breathe them out and breathe calm thoughts in. When you feel in control, communicate what has made you angry to your partner, boss, mother, child, or friend.

10 Learn to relax
Try different relaxation techniques, such as deep breathing, meditation, visualization, or aromatherapy. This section is packed with ideas!

OnTheSpot**StressSolutions**

Stress increases muscle tension, which heightens stress, and consequently leads to more muscle tension! To help break the cycle, relax and loosen up those tight spots in your body. When you are calm and relaxed, you look better, too. You can do these quick tension busters at any time, and almost anywhere.

UNCRAMP YOUR CALVES

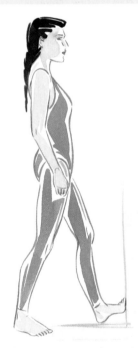 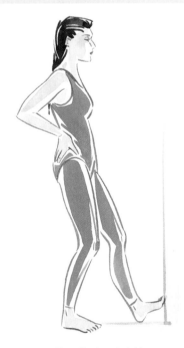

1 Remove shoes, stand up and face a wall, then place the ball of your left foot against the wall—the heel of your foot should not leave the floor.

2 Keep the leg straight as you press your hip in toward the wall. Hold for 10 seconds and relax. Change legs and do the same on the right foot.

FOR OVERWROUGHT WRISTS

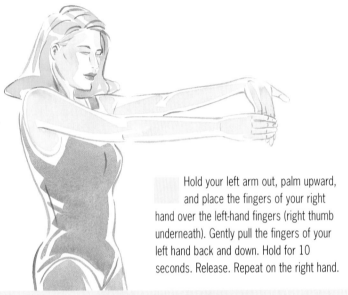

Hold your left arm out, palm upward, and place the fingers of your right hand over the left-hand fingers (right thumb underneath). Gently pull the fingers of your left hand back and down. Hold for 10 seconds. Release. Repeat on the right hand.

JAW RELAXER

Press your middle finger into the indentation at the top of the jaw line. To find the right spot, slide your middle finger about 1½ in (4 cm) from your left ear to your cheek and down to just above the jawbone. Press firmly for 1 minute. Repeat on the other side.

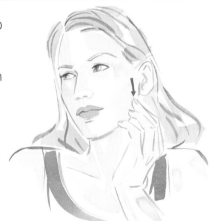

■ If you are using a keyboard most of the day, shake your wrists out regularly to relax them. Alternatively, roll a pencil up and down between your palm and your upper wrist. This may also help to prevent possible repetitive strain injury.

■ A good de-stressing technique for a stiff jaw is simply to open your mouth as wide as possible and hold it open for 5–10 seconds, then relax.

■ Try not to wear high-heel shoes all the time. It's bad for your back and posture and puts strain on your calf muscles. The muscles can tighten up, producing a stiff, uncomfortable feeling, including cramp. Stroke your calf muscles with your hand or with a small massage roller. This will improve the circulation and loosen the connecting tissue around the muscles.

SootheAway StressHeadaches

Tension headaches are felt as a diffuse pain over the top of your head or back of your neck, or as a tight band constricting your head. These unpleasant sensations are caused by a tightening of the muscles in your neck, scalp, and face, which puts pressure on blood vessels and nerves. Since tension headaches are caused by stress, the best way to avoid headaches is to relax and calm down. However, once a headache has taken hold, or when you feel the first twinges, try one of these simple on-the-spot solutions. The soothing action of a gentle head massage, for example, will relieve the muscle tension that so often precedes the headache and will help you to relax tense muscles. The beauty of this massage is that you can do it at home or at work.

RELAXING HEAD MASSAGE

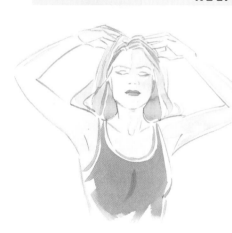

1 Place fanned fingertips on the crown of your head and press toward the back of your head in a slow, but firm, circular motion. Continue over your scalp and around your ears.

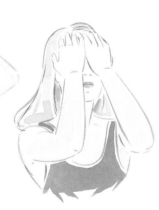

2 Cover your eyes with the palms of your hands. Breathe in and out deeply, concentrating hard on the rhythmic sound of your breathing. Hold the position for 1–2 minutes.

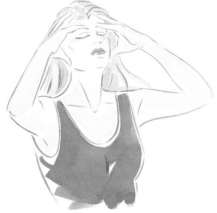

3 Hook your thumbs underneath your jaw and fan your fingers around the temples and forehead, pressing firmly. Release and repeat, working from the jawbone to the chin.

QUICK CALMERS

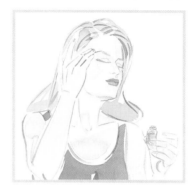

Massage a drop of neat lavender essential oil onto your temples. Or add lavender and peppermint oils in equal proportions, and mixed in a teaspoon (5 ml) of milk, to your bath.

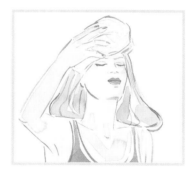

Apply an ice pack, or a pack of frozen peas wrapped in a clean cloth, to the back of your neck, temples, or forehead to help relieve head and neck pain and tension.

HELPFUL HEALTH TIPS

■ If you frequently suffer from headaches, keep track of them with a headache diary. Headaches can be caused by hormonal changes, the weather, poor posture, cigarette smoke (this increases carbon dioxide in the blood and reduces oxygen, leading to headaches), dehydration due to alcohol, allergies, or plain old anxiety. Try to isolate your personal headache triggers and avoid these situations.

■ You may not feel like it, but gentle exercise can help ease your headache. Not only does it allow you to release stress and pent-up emotions, it also improves blood circulation to the muscles. A burst of vigorous exercise also releases endorphins—the body's natural pain killers—into the body.

■ If you feel a sudden build-up of tension, take time out. Sit somewhere on your own—in the bathroom, where you can lock the door if necessary—and take at least 20 slow, deep breaths. Breathe in slowly through your nose, take the breath deep down, and exhale slowly through your mouth.

DeskStretchers

Sitting hunched over your computer or cradling the telephone between your shoulder and ear will give you a knotted neck and shoulders. In only 10 minutes you can stretch away the stress.

UNKNOT YOUR NECK

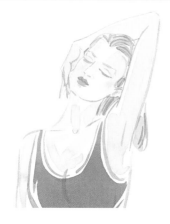

Raise your left arm in the air and curve it over the top of your head, resting your palm over your right ear. Let the weight of your arm gently pull your head to the left. Hold for 5–10 seconds. Release and repeat on the other side. Repeat 3 times each side.

UNBURDEN YOUR SHOULDERS

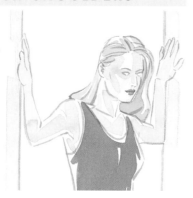

Stand in the center of a doorway with your feet together, your elbows bent, and your hands holding each side of the door frame. Keep your shoulders pressed down and lean forward, pushing your chest up and out. Hold for 10 seconds. Relax and repeat 5 times.

NECK AND SHOULDER STRETCH

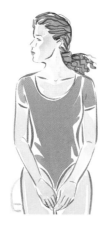

1 Sit upright in a chair and look straight ahead. Turn your head slowly to look to the left. Return to center. Turn your head slowly to the right, then return to center.

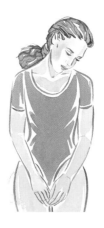

2 Gently allow your head to drop forward toward your left shoulder. Hold until you feel some of the tension release from your neck muscles.

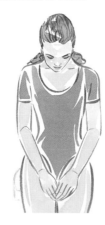

3 Then allow your head to roll slowly to the center, keeping your chin tucked into your chest.

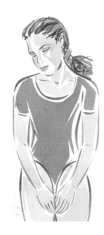

4 Roll your head around to your right shoulder and feel the stretch as before. Repeat the sequence 3 times.

TIPS

■ Shrugging your shoulders is an instant relaxer, and you can do it anywhere. Keep your arms at your sides and gently lift your shoulders up toward your ears. Stretch your shoulders as high as possible, then pull them down as far as possible. Repeat 5 times.

■ To relax a stiff neck, massage a couple of drops of lavender essential oil into your neck area and behind your ears.

■ If you make the same journey regularly, identify places on the route approximately 10 minutes apart. Remember to check your posture each time you pass one of your chosen landmarks. You can do this whether you are driving, walking, or on the train, or bus. You will be surprised how far your shoulders can creep up in just 10 minutes!

PressAwayStress

Acupressure, also known as shiatsu, is a system of treating disorders by pressing on the skin at precise points. It is based on the same theory as acupuncture—that the energy of life, known as chi, flows through the body along 14 channels called meridians. Each of the main meridians influences a major organ, which malfunctions if the flow of energy is disrupted. Pressing on the relevant point for 3–7 seconds restores the energy flow.

PRESS AND RELEASE

For a general feeling of wellbeing and contentment, press either side of the wrist just above the wrist bone. Use the thumb and index finger of the other hand.

When you have trouble sleeping, press the hollow just above the bony prominence on the inside of your ankle. Use the middle finger of one hand.

If your response to stress is comfort eating, press in the middle of the groove running from the nose to the top lip with the index finger of one hand. This can help beat the craving for an unhealthy snack.

TENSION HEADACHE

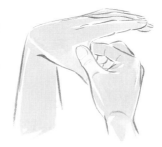

1 Pinch hard on the web of skin between the thumb and index finger. Next curl your hand into a fist and, with the other hand, pinch just below the little finger at the side.

2 With your thumb on the back of your wrist and index finger on your palm, press firmly on the back of the wrist in the middle.

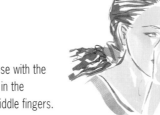

3 Press at the bridge of the nose with the thumb and ring finger. Press in the middle of the eyebrows with your middle fingers.

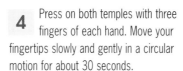

4 Press on both temples with three fingers of each hand. Move your fingertips slowly and gently in a circular motion for about 30 seconds.

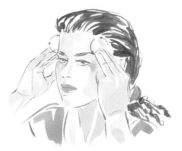

HELPFUL HEALTH TIPS

■ For menstrual pains, squeeze on each side of the ankle just above the bony area. Also press the inside of the leg about four finger-widths above the bony ankle area.

■ For tired eyes, press the outer sides of the top of nose—the point at the top of the nose and the inner corners of the eyes.

■ For tired feet, press a "line" along the middle of the big toe with the fingertips of one hand, supporting the toe with the fingers of the other hand.

■ To relieve fatigue, press on the top joint of your little finger.

Take Care

Bear in mind when doing acupressure squeezes that you are working on easing the symptoms. If these symptoms are recurrent and persistent, you should always seek the advice of a medical practitioner.

ThinkTranquility

Visualizing peaceful scenes and imagining wonderful scents and colors can promote a state of relaxation. Thinking positive thoughts when you are very relaxed may also influence your subconscious for the good and can help build your self-confidence. Take 10 minutes out of your day to create a feeling of calm and wellbeing.

SIX STEPS TO CALMING THOUGHTS

1 Lie down on a couch or bed
Make sure you are comfortable. Let your hands rest by your sides with palms up. Take a deep breath and release it slowly.

2 Tense and then relax your muscles
First focus on any tension in your feet. Clench your toes, then release and wriggle them. Work up through your legs, stomach, along your arms, fingers, and up your chest, tightening then relaxing your muscles. Release any tension in your shoulders and neck. Imagine the tightness in your face being soothed by gentle fingertips. Feel the tension ebb away through your scalp.

3 Breathe slowly and regularly
Concentrate on each breath. Each time everyday thoughts and worries intrude, focus back on your breathing. Tell yourself that you are becoming more and more relaxed. Close your eyes. Take four long deep breaths in and out, and let yourself relax completely.

4 Picture yourself at the top of a flight of stairs
Look down to the bottom of the stairs and see a stressfree haven waiting for you below. Use whatever image works for you—a beautiful beach, a peaceful garden, cool lakes and mountains, or some other favorite vacation spot.

5 Walk slowly down the stairs
As you walk down the stairs, tell yourself you are becoming more and more relaxed. If there is a specific cause of stress, use this stage to think positive thoughts about the resolution of your problem.

6 Enjoy your haven
When you reach the bottom of the stairs, walk into your haven. Really work at seeing and sensing all the details. If you imagine a beach, smell the sea and hear the gulls; in a garden, imagine touching and smelling the flowers. The more times you visit your haven, the more detailed you can make the scene. After 5 to 10 minutes, when you feel really relaxed, walk slowly back up the stairs. At the top, count to three, and open your eyes. Stretch, take several deep breaths, and get up slowly.

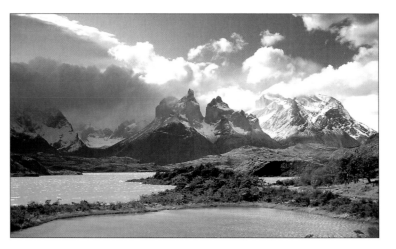

HELPFUL HEALTH TIPS

■ Read this six-step visualization into a tape recorder—or ask a friend with a calm voice to do it for you. That way you can lie back and listen to the instructions without any distractions.

■ Visualization and self-calming techniques can be used to help change bad habits. Use them to stop food cravings, or give up smoking. When you get to the stairway stage of the visualization, tell yourself that you can achieve what you want. If it is to stop smoking, for example, tell yourself "I will give up smoking." Imagine the smell of smoke spoiling your beautiful haven at the bottom of the stairs. See yourself throwing away the cigarettes as you walk down the stairs. See yourself happy and content in your haven without the need for cigarettes.

■ Keep a photograph of a peaceful, beautiful place in your purse or pocket. When you start to feel tense, take the picture out and focus on it for 5 minutes, breathing deeply.

TenQuick Visualizations

These quick visualizations will help to calm you and restore your sense of perspective. Use them when you are standing in line at the supermarket, when you are waiting for someone who is late, or when your car won't start! Whenever you are in a stressful situation where it is safe to "tune out" for a few minutes (not while you are driving!), try one of these instant vacations from stress.

ANYTIME, ANYWHERE

1 Stand in the sun
Picture yourself standing in a warm, sunny place. The sun's heat is relaxing all the tension and anger in your body. Breathe in the golden light. Let it fill your body. Breathe out black, angry thoughts. Let them dissolve in the sun's warmth.

2 Walk into the sun
Imagine walking slowly into the sun. Feel its heat and light power through your body dissolving any tension in your muscles.

3 Breathe in color
Imagine the air that you are breathing is a color. Choose yellow or orange if you are feeling depressed; blue or green if you feel angry. Breathe in the colored air. Breathe out gray or red air. Let your frustration or anger flow out with your breath.

4 Let problems float away
Picture your worries as balloons. Watch them float out of sight into a peaceful blue sky. As the balloons vanish, decide to go and do a completely different activity. Going for a walk would be great, but if that is not possible, tackle a different job or project.

5 Cut yourself loose
If it is a person causing you stress, cut yourself free of them in your mind. Imagine a pair of scissors cutting a cord between you. Concentrate on positive aspects—imagine having good times with this person, but also enjoying yourself without them.

6 Wild weather blows away worries
Picture yourself walking into a strong wind. The wind is blowing right through your mind and body and carrying away grievances, angers, and stress. Take deep breaths of the fresh air.

7 Let water soothe and relax you
Visualize yourself standing under a gentle waterfall in a peaceful, warm place. Hear the sound of the water falling down around you. Imagine the water washing away your stress.

8 Take a walk in your mind
See yourself walking away from crowded city streets onto a woodland trail. There is a breeze, the sun is warm, a stream runs beside the path. Smell the grass and see the color of the trees and flowers.

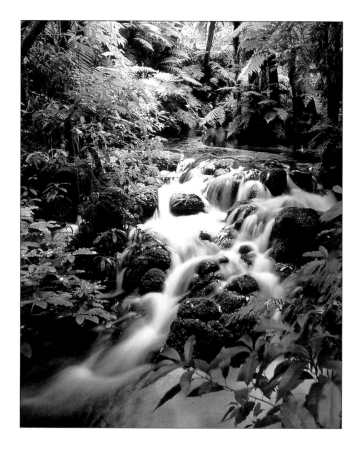

9 Enjoy a stress-busting activity—in your head
Visualize yourself dancing to loud music or imagine swimming in a warm lake. The activity can be anything from picking a beautiful bunch of flowers to skiing down a mountainside!

10 Get a sense of perspective
Picture yourself floating into the air, leaving your anxieties on the ground. They become smaller and less important. Float away from your stress until you reach a beautiful, calming scene to gaze down on.

Calming Scents

Aromatherapy is the therapeutic use of scented plant and flower-based essential oils for the prevention and cure of common health and beauty problems. Keep a selection of oils on hand for instant stress relief and relaxation.

POPULAR ESSENTIAL OILS

- **Chamomile** Calms and soothes the nervous system.
- **Clary sage** Eases depression, lessens anxiety, fear, and oversensitivity to others.
- **Frankincense** Promotes tranquility and calm.
- **Jasmine** Has an uplifting effect, alleviates anxiety.
- **Juniper** Helps ease depression and feelings of negativity.
- **Lavender** Helps relieve depression and insomnia.
- **Neroli** Eases shock and insomnia.
- **Rose** Harmonizes emotions and promotes inner calm.
- **Sandalwood** Calms, balances, and grounds.

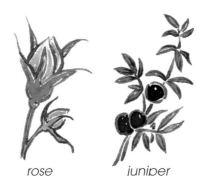

rose   *juniper*

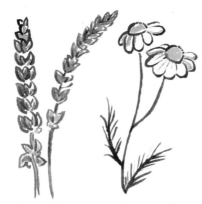

lavender   *chamomile*

HOW TO USE OILS

■ Most essential oils are too concentrated to use directly on the skin. But lavender and tea tree are sometimes used neat in tiny quantities for their healing and antiseptic qualities.

■ For massage, essential oils must be diluted in a carrier oil. Many purchased aromatherapy products come already mixed in oil, but it can be cheaper to mix your own. Combine 2, 3, or 4 essential oils, using two drops of each, with 2 teaspoons (10 ml) of a carrier oil. Sweet almond oil, avocado oil, evening primrose oil, or olive oil can be used as carrier oils. These quantities are enough for a neck-and-shoulder massage. Double the quantities for a full body massage.

■ For a fragrant bath, add up to 8 drops of a single oil, or a combination of up to four different oils, in a teaspoon (5 ml) of carrier oil or milk.

■ Wash as usual in the shower, then add a few drops of your chosen oil mixed with a teaspoon (5 ml) of carrier oil to a damp sponge and rub over your body. Inhale.

■ Add eight drops of oil to a basin of steaming water. Bend over the basin, cover your head with a towel, and inhale. Avoid steaming your face if you have very sensitive skin.

■ For an air-freshener, put 10 drops of essential oil into a plant spray containing cooled, boiled water. Do not spray on polished surfaces.

■ A ceramic aromatherapy diffuser holds water in a dish, to which you add three or four drops of oil. The water is heated with a votive candle and slowly evaporates, dispersing the scent of the oil. Essential oils are flammable, so keep the diffuser topped up with water.

HELPFUL HEALTH TIPS

■ To relieve tension try a combination of neroli, chamomile, jasmine, and sandalwood. Depression may be eased with jasmine, neroli, or rose.

■ Put a few drops of jasmine, chamomile, or lavender oil onto a tissue and inhale the vapors to help you sleep. Breathe slowly and deeply.

■ Rosemary is good to use when you have a cold or flu or feel generally run down. Mix with a teaspoon (5 ml) of carrier oil and use in a warm bath.

Take Care

Essential oils are powerful. Always keep them out of reach of children. Do not take internally unless you are being guided by a professional. Pregnant women are advised not to use clary sage. Those using clary sage or frankincense are advised not to drive or operate machinery after use.

ColorTherapy

In Eastern medicine the seven colors of the rainbow correspond to seven states, called "chakras." Each chakra is found at a particular point on the spine or head and is thought to control certain physical and emotional states. For example, color therapists use the color orange to treat problems, such as allergies, which are connected with a chakra at the small of the back. Without studying the technicalities of color therapy, you can use the basic principles to enhance your relaxation routines. Read the notes below and think about how you use color in your home, at work, and in the clothes you wear. Switch to energizing colors if you feel depressed. Choose calming colors if you feel anxious.

Indigo is cool and clarifying and helps create balance between people and their environments. It is used to treat emotional problems.

Violet helps harmonize the mind, body, and spirit. It can help alleviate insomnia and tension.

Blue represents love, truth, and communication. It is a relaxing, soothing color and helps to lower blood pressure, heart rate, and respiration. Blue is not recommended if you need more get up and go. It is also perceived as a conservative choice for clothes; wearing blue may inspire trust, but it could also make you seem lacking in creativity.

Green is the color of balance, calm, and compassion. It is uplifting, so it is helpful if you are tired, stressed, depressed, negative, angry, or tense. Green is good for headaches, too. A mixture of blue and green combines these colors' soothing and mood-enhancing qualities and is particularly relaxing and good for relieving tension.

Yellow is powerful and energizing. In color therapy, yellow represents wisdom, clear thinking, and self-knowledge. It can help if you are feeling mentally and emotionally low. In clothes, yellow is seen as fun and sunny, but sometimes tiresome and childish.

Orange is stimulating and is related to friendliness, creativity, sexuality, emotions, and intuition. Orange encourages a sense of self-worth and gives confidence. It is not recommended if you are dieting—it is said to encourage impulsive behavior, such as bingeing. Orange can help physical aches and pains, as well as muscular cramps.

Red warms the body, increases the heart rate, brain activity, and respiration. It is not recommended if you suffer from hypertension, high blood pressure, or asthma. Red clothes give you confidence, but do not promote harmony. Pink is a soothing color, the color of love and creativity.

■ Take a "color bath" to change your mood. Create red baths with berry herbal teas, yellow with chamomile tea, green with green or peppermint tea.

■ Seek out pleasant colors in the world around you. Plan your walk to work to go past gardens; buy yourself flowers for the home or office; keep colorful fruits and vegetables on display in your kitchen.

■ For instant color therapy, simply close your eyes and visualize the therapeutic color you need. Breathe deeply and concentrate on letting the color fill your body.

■ Replace your normal bedroom lightbulb with a colored one. Lie down, relax, and be bathed in your chosen color.

Meditation**ForCalm**

Meditation is a form of deep relaxation that allows your body to rest while your mind stays in a state of "relaxed alertness." Studies have shown that meditating regularly can substantially reduce stress levels. This is thought to be due to a decrease in the body's oxygen consumption as cell metabolism slows down and the brain's alpha waves, which are associated with relaxation, increase. The pulse and rate of breathing also slow down. Meditation has also been shown to help those who rely on alcohol to relieve anxiety.

MEDITATION METHOD

■ In a quiet room, sit cross-legged on the floor or on a firm chair. Check your back is straight and your shoulders relaxed. Rest your hands in your lap. Alternatively, lie on the floor with the palms of your hands up and your feet relaxed. Close your eyes.

■ Breathe deeply and evenly, as you imagine every part of your body relaxing. Work down from your scalp, relaxing each part of your body. Imagine a warm glow is traveling down through you.

■ Relax your mind and empty it of thoughts. Visualize unwanted thoughts as clouds and watch them float away.

■ You may find it helpful to have a "mantra"—a word that has no psychological associations (use a made-up word if you like) or a sound—and repeat it silently to yourself. Pay attention to the sound of the word, not its meaning.

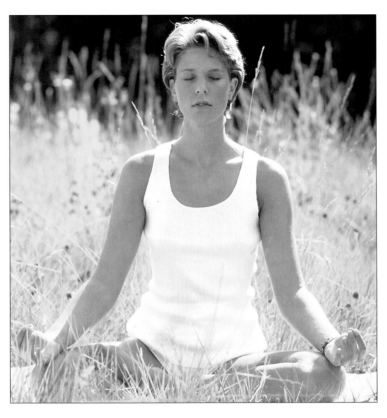

■ Concentrate on your breathing, feeling the air as it enters your nostrils and travels down to fill your lungs. As you breathe out, feel the air leaving your body. Try to breathe from your abdomen, not from your chest.

■ Meditate like this for a few minutes, twice a day. As you become more comfortable meditating, increase the time to 10 minutes or longer. At the end of your meditation time, stretch out, wait a minute or two to prevent yourself from becoming dizzy, and get up slowly.

HELPFUL HEALTH **TIPS**

■ Don't eat or drink for half an hour before meditating. You are likely to feel too full to be comfortable. But don't meditate if you're hungry either. You won't be able to concentrate, and a growling stomach could disrupt the calm.

■ Before you begin your meditation, turn the television and radio off, take the phone off the hook, shut the doors and windows, so there is as little external noise as possible, and tell your partner or family that you do not want to be disturbed for 10 minutes.

■ You need to get rid of your negative emotions to relax fully. If you are angry with someone, you need to discuss why and sort it out. Alternatively, sit and write a letter explaining why you are angry or frustrated. This should help you work through the emotion until you get the chance to talk it through.

Healing Touches

Instinctively we rub and massage painful parts of our bodies. Not surprisingly, touch therapies have been used for centuries to treat aches and pains. Massage works on two levels—it helps to relieve the stress that causes ailments such as headaches, stomachaches, mild back pain, and insomnia, and it is effective in easing the symptoms of these problems when they do occur. A brisk self-massage can also increase your energy levels, especially if you use an uplifting aromatherapy oil, such as jasmine or rosemary. Use soothing oils, such as chamomile or lavender, for a relaxing massage. Always mix undiluted essential oils with a carrier oil before putting them on the skin.

FACE REFRESHER

1 Give yourself a quick facial massage to relieve tension. Gently press with your fingertips around the under part of the eye sockets, working from the outer edge toward the nose. Then tap very lightly around the eye area using your ring fingers to reduce any eye puffiness.

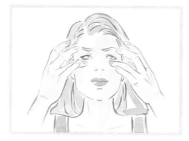

2 Starting with the center of the forehead and working out toward the hairline, press across the brow with your fingertips. Repeat several times.

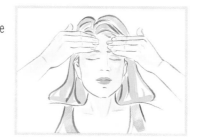

■ Never pour massage oil directly onto the skin. Pour a small amount into the palm of one hand and warm it between your palms.

■ When you massage your skin, imagine waves of heat passing through your fingers into your body. This increases the effectiveness of a relaxing massage.

■ To relax your eyes after driving a long distance or staring at a computer screen, rub your hands together until your palms feel warm. Close your eyes and cup your palms over them with your fingers on your forehead. Let the warmth from your palms sink into your skin.

ENERGY BOOSTING

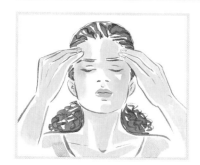

1 Close your eyes and place the fingertips of both hands on your forehead. Rhythmically pat over your face with your fingertips in a fast and energetic motion to help wake you up.

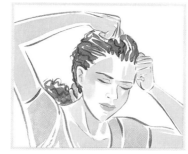

2 Clench your fists loosely and gently knead all over your head to help stimulate the circulation. Then unclench your fists and with open, relaxed hands, gently "slap" your head.

3 Raise your left leg slightly and pummel your thigh and buttocks with loose fists. Keep the movements vigorous and energetic. Work down the length of your leg, then repeat on your right thigh.

4 Sit down with your right foot resting on your left thigh. Press the point on the center of your sole just below the ball of the foot for 10 seconds to help increase energy.

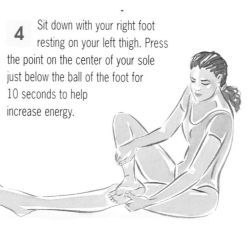

Head-and-toe Massage

Focusing on treating the head and feet can be the fastest route to relaxation. The neck is a critical junction between the head and the body. Massaging the neck muscles prevents shoulder and upper backache as well as tension headaches.

A 10-minute foot rub revitalizes your whole body. To massage your own feet, rest one foot on the opposite thigh if you are sitting. If you prefer to lie down, keep one leg bent and rest the other foot on your raised thigh. Work on one foot at a time.

NECK AND SHOULDERS

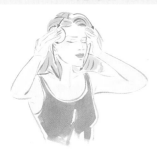

1 Starting at the top of the scalp, use your fingertips to rub gently but firmly in small circular movements working down toward your neck.

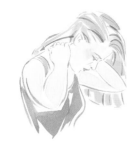

2 Use your fingertips to press firmly on muscles on both sides of the top of the spine. Slowly move your fingers outward around the neck.

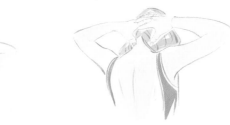

3 With your fingertips, press firmly on any tension spots at the top of your neck. Hold for a few seconds. Pinch the flesh along the shoulders.

4 Fan out clasped fingers over the back of your head. Press your thumbs into the dips at the base of skull. Hold for 10–20 seconds. Relax and repeat.

FREE YOUR FEET

Hold each toe in turn with the fingers and thumb of one hand. Move the toe in a circular motion at the base. Then grip the base of each toe between your thumb and index finger and pull to stretch it. Massage the bottom of your feet by raking the knuckles of your clenched fist slowly from heel to toe. Hold one foot in both hands. Press your fingertips into the sole, then slide them toward the sides. Repeat the sequence for increased relaxation.

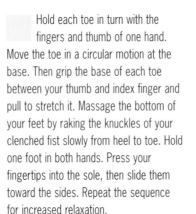

INSTANT INVIGORATOR

For an instant de-stressing and invigorating effect, hold your left foot with your left hand and with your right hand firmly stroke your knuckles down the sole, from heel to toe, several times (right). Then lightly "karate" chop the arch with the side of your right hand. Do this 5–10 times. Repeat on your right foot.

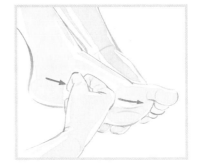

HELPFUL HEALTH TIPS

■ If your feet feel hot and sweaty, massage them with a blend of 2 drops of peppermint and 2 drops of tea tree essential oils mixed with a carrier oil.

■ Roll a golf ball or rolling pin around the sole of your foot for a quick foot massage. Alternatively, massage your foot by rubbing the sole along the crossbar of the chair or table.

■ Reflexologists believe that each part of the foot represents part of the body—toes are the head and neck, the heel is the lower body. Tender areas of the foot represent a problem area elsewhere in your body and can be treated by treating the foot. For a sore neck, work on the inner side and base of your big toe. To work the spine, press all along the inside edge of each foot, from the big toe to the heel, following the line of the arch of the foot.

Massage MadeEasy

Massage soothes the body and mind, and is thought to stimulate the flow of endorphins (opiate-like substances) through the body. Massage also speeds up the elimination of waste toxins, stimulates the circulation, and eases tense muscles. Persuade a friend to give you a 10-minute massage when you are feeling stressed. Return the favor when he or she is under pressure.

BASIC MASSAGE TECHNIQUES

Traditional massage consists of three basic strokes: effleurage (stroking), petrissage (kneading), and tapotement (striking). The first two are the safest and simplest to do at home.

Stroking is a firm, but gentle, continuous movement down the body using the whole hand. Kneading—squeezing and rolling the fleshy areas of the body—is a deeper stroke. You can knead quite hard with both your thumbs and the heel of your hand. Striking consists of cupping, pummeling, flicking, and slapping the fleshy parts of the body.

A massage can be stimulating or soothing. It's a matter of varying the intensity and type of strokes used and choosing an appropriate aromatherapy oil (see page 88).

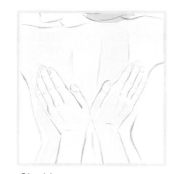

Stroking

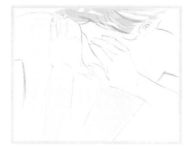

Kneading

NECK AND BACK MASSAGE

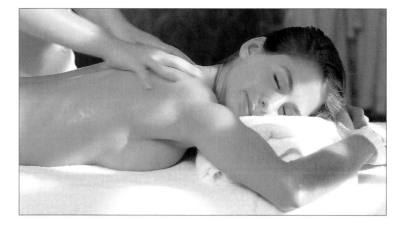

1   In a warm, quiet room, make a soft bed of towels on the floor. The person being massaged should lie face down on the towels in a comfortable position.

2   Remove jewelry and warm your hands. Rub a few drops of massage oil between your hands (see page 88). Rest them on the person you are massaging to establish initial contact.

3   Try to maintain contact with the skin so the massage feels like a continuous movement. Stopping and starting breaks the flow and makes the massage less relaxing.

4   Start with stroking movements. Begin at the neck and move to the shoulders and back. Pay attention to any areas of knotted muscles—you will soon learn to recognize them.

5   Knead the muscles gently, then smooth the areas around them with stroking motions. If your hands get tired at any point, continue stroking.

6   Slow the rhythm and pressure of the massage as you come to the end. Finish by resting your hands in one position on the back for about a minute. Let your friend rest for a while, then have him or her get up slowly.

TIPS

■ An oiled body loses heat quickly, so always put warm soft towels over exposed areas that you are not massaging. All the relaxing effects of your massage will go to waste if your massage partner is cold.

■ Turn the lights down low, play some soft background music, and burn incense sticks or an aromatherapy candle to create a soothing atmosphere.

■ Keep a bowl of oil in a warm dish by your side during the massage. Use extra oil to massage dry areas of skin, for example, around the elbows.

Take Care

Do not massage anyone suffering from acute back pain, or fighting an infection or contagious disease, or who has a temperature or any other serious medical complaint. Some essential oils should not be used by a pregnant woman, who is either giving or receiving a massage—consult a qualified aromatherapist or medical practitioner.

Deep**Breathing**

The art of breathing correctly is central to the promotion of relaxation and the maintenance of youthful looks. If you are not breathing as efficiently as you could be, your skin tone will be the first thing to suffer. Seven percent of the oxygen you take in is used by the skin, so the less fresh oxygen you take into your body, the less there is for your skin.

BREATHING TECHNIQUE

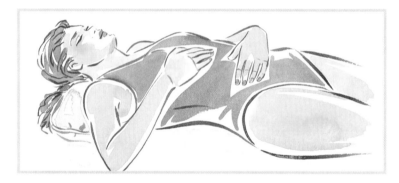

1 Lie flat on your back with a small pillow under your neck. Place one hand on your abdomen. Breathe in slowly through your nose, imagining you are sending breath to below your navel. Your stomach should start to swell.

2 Let the breath fill the rest of your stomach and expand your rib cage. Rest your hand on one side of your rib cage to feel it move up.

3 Continue to let this breath fill the upper part of your chest area. The inhalation process should take around 5 seconds.

4 Hold your breath for 5 seconds then start to breathe out, contracting your lower abdomen gently to move the air upward. The exhalation process should take about 5 seconds. Rest a few seconds. Repeat the steps.

1 Stand with your arms by your sides. Take a minute to feel balanced. Make sure your feet are slightly apart and parallel to each other. Check your shoulders are down, your arms and hands relaxed at your sides. Then take a long breath in through your nose.

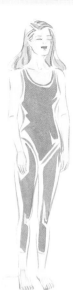

2 Raise your shoulders up toward your ears, clench your fists, and stand on tiptoe. Tense your body harder and harder as you do this. Keep your stomach muscles tightly pulled in as this will also help you to balance.

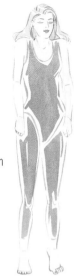

3 Hold your breath and slowly lower your heels to the floor. At the same time, loosen your shoulders and let them drop, too.

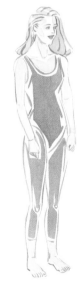

4 Unclench your fists and breathe out slowly through your nose. Feel the heavy weight of your tension leave your body through your palms as you exhale. Take a few normal breaths and then repeat the sequence. Do this up to 10 times.

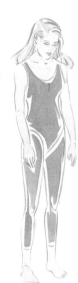

HELPFUL HEALTH **TIPS**

■ Concentrate on breathing regularly and evenly in stressful situations. This will slow down your heart rate and make you feel more in control. Concentrate on speaking slowly, too. This will help you to feel and appear more relaxed.

■ Another quick relaxation tip is to sigh loudly and as deeply as you can, then take in a good breath of fresh air.

■ Stand in front of a mirror and watch your shoulders as you breathe. They should not move at all if you are breathing deeply and properly—your abdomen should be the only thing moving.

■ Try alternate nostril breathing to wake yourself up and improve your concentration. Close your right nostril with your right thumb and breathe in deeply through your left nostril. Close your left nostril with your right index finger and breathe out through your right nostril. Now reverse the sequence, breathing in through the right nostril and out through the left. Continue this for a couple of minutes.

Hand&Foot StressBusters

You can release a lot of stress and tension by doing these simple hand and foot exercises. The best thing about hand stretches is that you can do them almost anywhere—at work, stuck in a traffic jam, on a train, or sitting watching television. These routines will also help to keep your hands and feet flexible, and strengthen and firm the muscles in your arms and legs. A lot of benefits for a little effort!

HANDY HINTS

1 Sit comfortably but upright in a chair or cross-legged on the floor. Straighten your arms out to your sides and spread your fingers as wide apart as you can. Hold for 10 seconds. Relax your hands and arms. Repeat 6 times.

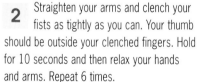

2 Straighten your arms and clench your fists as tightly as you can. Your thumb should be outside your clenched fingers. Hold for 10 seconds and then relax your hands and arms. Repeat 6 times.

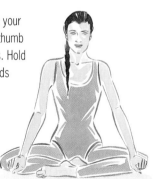

FINGER EXERCISES

1 Use your right hand to grip each finger in turn on your left hand. Pull gently, but firmly, for 5 seconds. Let your hand slide up the finger to release it. Do all the fingers, then switch hands.

2 Beginning with the little finger of your right hand and moving one finger at a time, stretch each finger down to touch the base of the palm. Stretch the thumb across to touch the little finger. Repeat 5 times and then do the left hand.

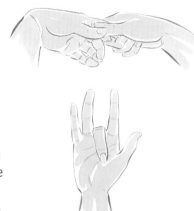

FOOTWORK

1 Sitting on the floor, and with your legs straight out in front of you, point your toes. Stretch the top of your feet as much as you can. Hold for about 5 seconds, then relax. Repeat 5 times.

2 Bend one foot toward you and hold for 5 seconds, then relax. Bend the other foot toward you, hold, and relax. Repeat with alternate feet 5 times. Finish by wiggling and stretching your toes as much as you can. They may not move very much at first, but over time you should get more movement.

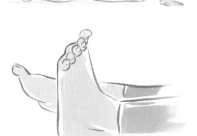

HELPFUL HEALTH TIPS

■ To relax your feet after standing all day, add up to 4 drops of a favorite essential oil—lavender or sandalwood is a good choice—mixed with a teaspoon (5 ml) of carrier oil, to a large bowl of hot water. Soak your feet for 10 minutes.

■ Circle your wrists and ankles clockwise, then counter-clockwise, several times a day. This will help to keep your joints flexible.

■ Keep little jars of hand cream all around the house and in your office desk. Use the cream to massage your hands whenever they feel cold or when your skin feels dry. Give your feet the same treatment after a bath or before you go to bed.

Stress-relieving Stretches

Muscular tension is the body's natural response to stress. The shoulders, neck, and lower back tend to be the most stress-prone sites. This simple series of stretches targets the tension hotspots in your body. Change into loose, comfortable clothes and use a mat or towel to lie on.

FULL BODY STRETCH

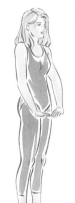

1 Stand with your hands in front of you at the tops of your thighs, with fingers pointing toward each other and palms down.

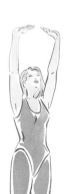

2 Move your arms forward and upward while breathing in slowly through your nose. Hold your arms above your head, pushing your palms toward the ceiling, pulling your elbows close to your ears.

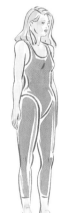

3 Hold the stretch and breathe out through your mouth. Slowly lower your arms down to your sides. Repeat the steps 10 times and build up to more repetitions.

LEG LIGHTENER

1 Sit cross-legged on the floor with your back straight. Bend your legs in front of you and press the soles of your feet together. Hold onto your ankles and use your elbows to press your thighs and knees down toward the floor. Hold for 20 seconds. Repeat.

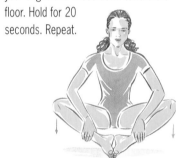

2 Lie on your back. Bend your knees so your feet are flat on the floor. Raise your left leg to your chest, holding it behind the calf. Stretch (do not straighten) the raised leg and pull it toward you. Hold for 10—20 seconds. Relax. Change legs.

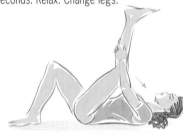

STRETCH THEN RELAX

Lie flat on your back, looking at the ceiling, and bring your knees into your chest. Wrap your arms around your legs for support. Gently roll your head to the right, then bring it very slowly back to the starting position. Let your head roll to the left. Bring it slowly back to center.

Put your feet on the floor and slide your legs out straight. Put your arms at your side, palms up. Relax fully for 5 minutes, breathing slowly and deeply.

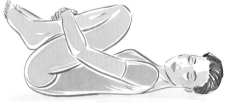

HELPFUL HEALTH TIPS

■ If you have time, warm up before you start the stress-relieving stretches on this page. March in place, run up and down the stairs, or dance for a few minutes. This will raise your body temperature and help release any pent-up anger.

■ Breathe slowly as you perform each stretch, breathing in through your nostrils, pausing before you breathe out, then slowly releasing all the air in your lungs and pausing before filling your lungs with air again. As you do each stretch, keep telling yourself you are relaxing and slowing down.

■ Firm feet will allow the rest of your body to relax and move more freely. When standing, keep your weight on your heels so you can spread your toes out wide and the arches of your feet feel strong and springy. This allows your spine to straighten and lengthen. Relax your shoulders and arms and feel your head balance naturally on top of your spine.

Spine Thrillers

These stretches may be familiar to you if you have ever been to a yoga class. Yoga is the perfect antidote to stress, combining as it does mental tranquility with physical fitness and spiritual awareness. Try these gentle poses, which have been specially selected to ease and strengthen your back.

THE SPINE TWIST

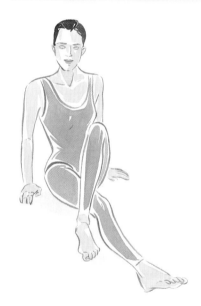

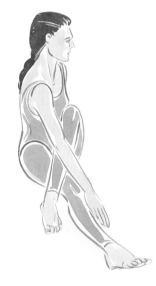

1 Sit with your legs stretched out in front of you, palms on the floor. Lift your left leg and place your foot on the far side of your right knee. Slowly turn your body to the left and reach toward your right ankle with your right hand.

2 Place your left hand behind you, palm down, trying to keep your back straight. Each time you breathe out, twist farther to the left. Stop when you feel stretched and hold for 10 seconds. Relax then repeat on the other side.

CAT STRETCH

1 Get down on all fours, your hands directly underneath your shoulders, hips over knees. Breathe slowly, trying to make your back as level as possible. Let your head and neck relax down.

2 Slowly push your spine up toward the ceiling, tucking your chin into your chest. Feel a stretch along your spine and shoulders. Do not push the stretch if you feel any discomfort. Hold for about 10 seconds.

3 Slowly bring your head up and push your spine down so your back is as concave as possible. Hold for about 10 seconds, then make your back level and relax your head and neck. Repeat the sequence several times.

COBRA

Lie on your stomach with your forehead on the floor. Put your hands palms down under your shoulders. Push your arms up and stretch your head up. Hold for about 10 seconds, then relax down. Repeat several times.

HELPFUL HEALTH

TIPS

■ If you enjoy stretching and calming exercises, look for a local yoga class to attend. It is an ideal form of exercise for all ages and degrees of fitness.

■ Stretch out and move around as much as possible during the day. This will stop tension from accumulating in your spine. Slumping at your desk, long periods of sitting down, poor posture, and feeling stressed can all take their toll on your back, so get stretching!

■ In yoga, breathing is considered the life-force of an individual's being, affecting emotional and spiritual harmony. Breathe evenly and deeply throughout the yoga stretches. Concentrate on breathing out for longer than you breathe in since this will help you to relax more.

Take Care

Do not push yourself into any position that feels uncomfortable or where you might lose your balance. If at any point you feel dizzy or faint, stop and relax.

EssentialDailyRelaxation

Relaxation is a skill. You have to learn how to do it and you need to practice regularly. The only equipment you need for this routine are comfortable clothes and a towel or mat to lie on. Aim to do the relaxer every day—when you get home from work, after a journey, or before bed. It is also beneficial to do this sequence after stretching.

REST AND RESTORE ROUTINE

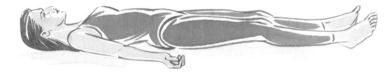

1 Lie on your back in a quiet, dimly lit room. Close your eyes. Let your feet flop outward and your arms fall away from the body, palms facing the ceiling. Breathe deeply and gently. Concentrate on your chest rising and falling as you breathe in and out. Make an effort to slow your breathing down. Screw up your face muscles, then relax them. Imagine that your skin is so relaxed that all the lines on your face are ironed out and your skin is slipping down toward the floor.

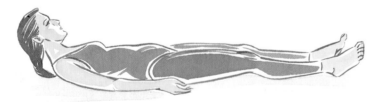

2 Press your shoulders into the floor. Hold for 10 seconds, relax and repeat. Lift your head off the floor without straining your neck, lengthen the back of the neck, and gently put your head down. Check your jaw and neck muscles are relaxed.

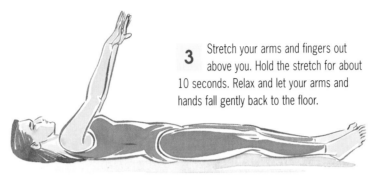

3 Stretch your arms and fingers out above you. Hold the stretch for about 10 seconds. Relax and let your arms and hands fall gently back to the floor.

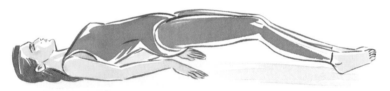

4 Hold in your stomach and lift your buttocks off the floor, without straining your lower back, then let them back down. Feel your spine stretch gently and relax. Keeping your legs together, stretch your legs and toes. Hold for 10 seconds, then relax, letting your feet fall open. If any part of your body still feels tense, repeat the sequence.

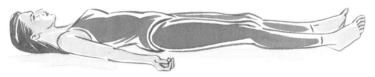

5 Stay in this relaxed pose for up to 10 minutes. Concentrate on your breathing whenever day-to-day worries enter your mind. Before you get up, roll onto your side and stay there for a minute. Get up slowly and carefully.

HELPFUL HEALTH TIPS

■ A traditional relaxation pose is shown here, but some people find it uncomfortable to lie flat on the floor. Try the sequence lying on your bed or use one of the alternative relaxation positions shown on page 99.

■ You may find you get cold quickly when you are fully relaxed. Have a throw or blanket handy to pull over you. You need to be warm to relax fully.

■ To help combat tension even more, burn a relaxing aromatherapy oil such as lavender or chamomile while you do relaxation routines. See page 88 for further information on aromatherapy.

■ A daily form of complete physical and mental relaxation will clear your mind and help to relieve recurrent backaches and headaches. It can also lower blood pressure and keep a number of physical complaints at bay.

RelaxInComfort

To relax fully, you must be comfortable. Lying flat on the floor to relax, as shown on the previous page, doesn't suit everybody. If your back aches, do the lower back soother before you lie flat. If you can't breathe freely lying flat, don't hesitate to put pillows beneath your head or beneath your back and head. This will help to relax your throat and jaw muscles. Or try one of these alternative relaxation positions. You may find 10 minutes relaxing in one of these poses is the perfect end to a busy day.

LOWER BACK SOOTHER

1 Lie flat on your back with your knees bent and your feet flat on the floor. Lift your buttocks just off the floor and press your lower back onto the floor. Lower your buttocks slowly.

2 Bring your knees up toward your chest and clasp your arms around them. Gently rotate your knees clockwise several times. Repeat the rotations in a counter-clockwise direction. Relax back into the starting position. Let your legs slide out straight and go into the relaxation routine on page 98.

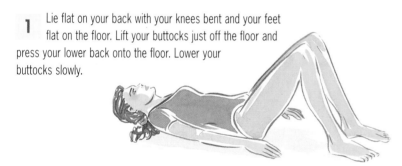

LEG AND BACK RELAXER

Select a chair with a flat seat. Put a pillow on the seat for extra comfort. Lie on the floor with your feet and calves supported by the chair. Try to position your thighs at right angles to the floor. Tense and relax your muscles—starting with your feet and working your way up to your head. Close your eyes and relax for up to 10 minutes.

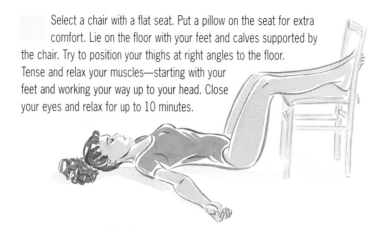

DRAIN AWAY STRESS

1 Lie flat on your back, leaning your fully extended legs and backs of heels against the wall. If you are fairly flexible, you should be able to place your legs flush against the wall, but if you are not, don't worry—put your legs at a comfortable angle to the wall. Your buttocks should rest comfortably on the floor.

2 Position your arms close by your sides with your elbows tucked into the body. "Roll" your shoulders under so your shoulder blades lie flat. Push your elbows and head flat against the floor and feel your chest lift slightly as you draw your shoulder blades down. Extend the back of your neck. Pull your stomach in.

3 Place the heels of your hands over your eyes, fanning your fingers out. At the end of each breath, feel your body relax and the tension drain out of you. Continue for 5 minutes.

HELPFUL HEALTH TIPS

■ After relaxing, don't just jump up. Bring your breathing back to normal if you have been taking deep breaths and open your eyes. Roll over onto your right side with your knees bent. Stay like that for a minute before getting up slowly.

■ Visualize something calm while you are relaxing if thoughts and worries keep popping into your mind. A simple, but effective technique for winding down when you're feeling tense is to imagine a relaxing and beautiful place in your mind, say a beach or a mountaintop. Imagine the view, the sounds, the smells of the place as you slowly begin to feel more relaxed and in control. For more information on visualization see pages 86 and 87.

■ Play some gentle, soothing music, such as dolphin, whale, or water music. Use earphones to block out all outside noise.

Stressfree Home

Your home should be a haven—a place where you can shut the door and enjoy life free from tension and anxiety. For the most part, home is a retreat from the stresses and strains of the day, but it can also be the source of tensions—arguing over who does the chores, having to cook a meal every night, feeling the house is never as clean as you would like it. Here are some quick ideas for stressproofing your home.

FIVE TIPS FOR A CALM HOME

1 Follow the 10-minute rule

If there are tasks around the house or yard that you have put off doing, do them for just 10 minutes. Set the kitchen timer or an alarm clock. Once you have started, you may well decide to spend longer. Having a huge clearout or cleaning something really dirty can be enjoyable! It's getting started that's the hard part. If you don't want to carry on after 10 minutes—fine. You have made a start and can do another 10 minutes another day.

2 Color your mood

Use color to change the mood of your home. Blue, for example, is soothing. Studies have shown that it can help calm hyperactive children. Make up for the lack of natural light in winter by adding accents of "sunnier" colors, such as yellows, golds, and oranges. An appropriately colored throw placed over the couch can be positioned in much less than 10 minutes! For more information on color therapy, see page 89.

3 Learn about Feng Shui

The ancient Chinese art of Feng Shui is a way of promoting harmony in your life by adjusting the style and layout of the rooms you inhabit. Clutter is thought to block the positive energy in your life, so clear out piles of old papers, magazines, clothes you never wear, and things you never use. Feng Shui recommends that you avoid having shelves above your work desk—they create a sense of oppression and increase levels of negative energy. If you find these ideas helpful, there are many books on Feng Shui that will tell you more.

4 Discover the sense of scents

Good smells such as fresh-baked bread, fresh-brewed coffee, and flowers make your home a more pleasant, relaxing place to live in. Aromatherapy oils smell great, and they can also influence people's moods. Burn a little geranium oil with a hint of melissa oil during a dinner party. This combination will both invigorate and relax, creating a good atmosphere. Citrus oils go well with spicy foods. Pine, cedarwood, and frankincense evoke the holiday season.

5 Ensure stressfree sleep

Your bedroom should be one room where you have absolute peace and relaxation. Try to keep it free from junk and associations of work-based stress. If you have to work in your bedroom, use a screen to divide your bed from your work area.

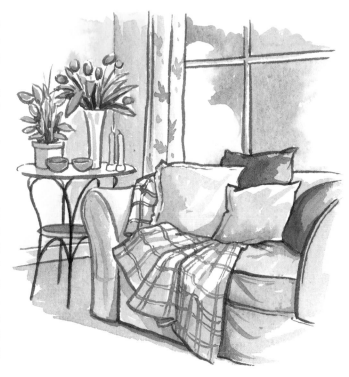

ArriveRelaxed

Stress isn't confined to the home or the workplace. Traveling, with all its potential frustrations and difficulties, can be a big stress inducer. Here are some simple solutions to the problems of traffic and transportation.

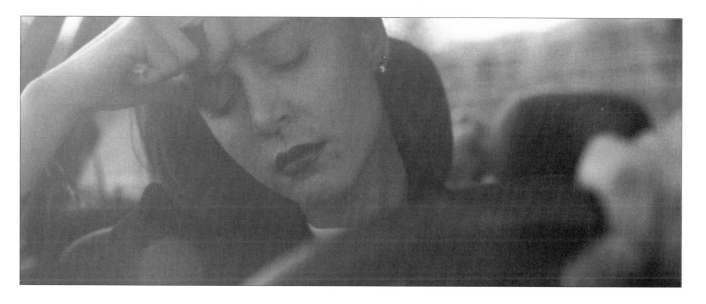

TEN TOP TRAVEL TIPS

1 Relax before you leave
Before a long journey, relax by taking a bath with a few drops of ginger, lavender, and peppermint essential oils mixed with a teaspoon (5 ml) of carrier oil or milk added to the water.

2 Fear of flying?
Before take-off and during the flight, do the hand exercises on page 95 and give yourself a soothing hand massage, using circular movements of the thumb of the opposite hand over the palm.

3 For blocked ears on planes
Make small circular movements with your fingertips to the front of the ears just above the jawbone. Then place your index fingers behind each ear, keeping the remaining fingers in front. Make slow circular counter-clockwise movements.

4 To prevent jet lag
Inhale ylang ylang essential oil. Drink fresh fruit and vegetable juices before you leave for a blast of vitamins. Do the stretches on pages 98 and 99 before bed to make sure you sleep soundly.

5 To stop motion sickness
Press on the center of your wrist for 3–7 seconds. Ginger supplements and ginger herbal tea may also stop you from feeling nauseous.

6 Stay calm while driving
Keep small bottles of relaxing aromatherapy oils in your purse. Put 10 drops on a tissue and inhale if delays or other drivers make you angry and tense. Deep breathing will also calm you. Breathe out for longer than you breathe in to slow your heart rate.

7 Stay alert
When driving long distances, stay alert by squeezing the middle of the palm—this acupressure point helps to stimulate and create energy. Inhale invigorating essential oils such as basil or rosemary. Play music and open the window. If you get very tired, the only safe answer is to take a rest break.

8 De-stress your neck and shoulder muscles
Sit with your spine upright and your shoulders as relaxed as possible. Slowly let your head drop toward your right shoulder as far as it can comfortably go, return to the center, and let it drop slowly to the left. Repeat 5 times.

9 Deal with delays
If you get stressed out by travel delays, try the simple stretches on pages 82 and 84. Alternatively, use one of the visualizations on page 87 to help distract you from your stressful situation. Always carry a book or magazine to read so you have something to do.

10 Freshen up
If you can, go and freshen up—wash your face, brush your teeth, and put on some makeup and perfume to help yourself feel human again.

5

LookGood

Being **Beautiful**

need not be dependent on how much time you spend in beauty salons or health clubs, or on how much money you have to lavish on fancy skin creams or expensive makeup. The best way to enhance your appearance and glow with good health is to treat your body well—by exercising it, feeding it the right "fuel," learning how to relax, and taking care of your skin and hair. Ten minutes is all you need to enjoy each of the beauty treatments explained here. They are easy, economical, and use everyday, inexpensive ingredients. Prop these pages open by your mirror and give yourself a well-deserved 10-minute treat!

Some of the most beautiful women in the world insist that their best beauty "secret" is water—simply drinking 6 to 8 glasses a day of filtered or bottled water. That's certainly one tip everyone can find the time and money to try! Undoubtedly these lovely women also stick to a health regime that could benefit us all: eating a healthy,

EASE balanced diet full of fresh fruit and vegetables, and exercising regularly. Many of these women also treat the outside of their bodies with simple, but effective, natural beauty methods: regular massage, facial exercises, using water to hydrate and pep up their skin, and using natural ingredients such as vegetable oils and vitamin E to moisturize their bodies.

In these days of hi-tech cosmetic

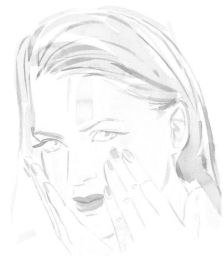

formulae and treatments, it is comforting to know that many expensive beauty solutions are just prettily packaged versions of age-old beauty recipes—with chemicals added to make them keep longer. You will soon

SIMPLE discover that most essential beauty ingredients can be found in your kitchen or bathroom. By preparing your own lotions and potions, you will not only save money, you will also know exactly what you are putting on your face and body, and so cut out many unwanted chemicals and perfumes.

To really look good you need to eat well, stimulate your circulation through exercise,

moderate your alcohol intake, quit smoking, get enough good-quality sleep, learn to unwind and get rid of stress, and try out some

LIFESTYLE of the natural beauty treatments in the pages that follow. Recognize that treating your skin and body with care will pay enormous dividends throughout your life. You are never too young or too old to look more beautiful.

Take Care

When trying a new skin care treatment, whether purchased or one you have made yourself, it is advisable to check for an allergic reaction or skin irritation. Do a patch test by dabbing a little of the product on your wrist or behind your ears and leaving for 24 hours. Always check with a dermatologist if you have an allergic reaction or skin irritation.

PerfectSkinForLife

Whatever type of skin you have, and whatever its condition, there are some simple steps that you can take today—and everyday—to improve its feel and appearance.

TEN WAYS TO CARE FOR YOUR SKIN

1 Eat right
No amount of beauty products can help your skin if you are not getting the right nutrients. A diet rich in fresh foods and low in processed and refined foods will improve the condition of your skin.

2 Drink more water
Skin experts tend to be dismissive about the powers of water, but women with beautiful skin swear by it. Aim to drink 6–8 large glasses a day.

3 Try not to frown
A miserable face certainly draws attention to your wrinkles! And frowning, furrowing, or wrinkling up your face is one of the surest ways to get lines. Make an effort not to furrow your face!

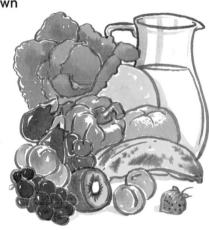

4 Breathe deep
Your skin needs to breathe. Instead of taking shallow breaths from the top of your chest, practice taking deep breaths to oxygenate the whole body. Check out the Deep Breathing on page 94.

5 Get an exercise glow
If you think your skin looks better after a good walk, you are right. When you exercise, oxygen surges to every cell in your body, blood circulation is improved, and your skin takes on a healthy glow.

6 Relax and look lovely
Stress is a big barrier to looking good. It causes you to tense your facial muscles, frown, and furrow your brow. It also tends to disrupt sleep patterns and may cause tension headaches and other ailments, making you feel and look ill. See Section 4—Calm & Relax for stress-beating tactics.

7 Sleep your way to super skin
Skin cells regenerate while you sleep and sound restorative sleep has an enhancing effect on your skin. Studies have shown that disrupted sleep may be linked to excessively dry skin or acne flare-ups. See page 125 for a checklist of ways to beat insomnia and improve your sleeping patterns.

8 Take care in the sun
Sun damage is probably the worst culprit for prematurely aging skin. Sunbathe in moderation and never between noon and 3 p.m. Always wear a highly protective sunblock. Use moisturizers and foundations containing SPFs, so your skin (including the backs of your hands) is protected daily. Wear a hat to protect your face and neck.

9 Keep up your cleansing routine
Poor cleansing allows bacteria to grow and sebum (the skin's natural oil) to accumulate causing blackheads, whiteheads, and pimples.

10 Treat your skin type right
Regular skin treatments, such as face masks, exfoliants, and facial oils, chosen to suit your skin, are not an indulgence. They really can improve its condition. Check out the following pages for ideas!

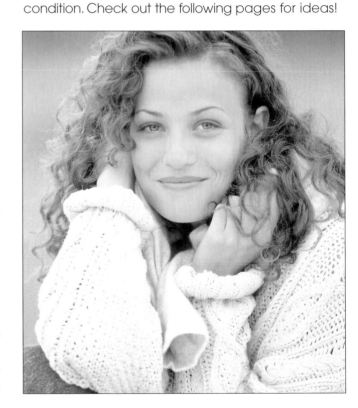

NormalSkinCare

You may be the lucky possessor of "normal" skin. If you don't have any special problems—no oiliness, dryness, or pimples, and your skin is generally soft, smooth, and supple—then you certainly are. But just because your skin is problem-free, doesn't mean it can't be brighter, clearer, and healthier looking. Your skin type can change, too—so start taking care of it now and be alert to changes.

FLORAL AND HERBAL STEAM

1 Clean your face with your normal cleanser. Fill a bowl with boiling water and add 1–2 drops of geranium, lavender, or rose essential oil, or pour boiling water over a handful of dried lavender, fresh elderflower, and/or marigold heads.

2 Put a towel over your head and the bowl. Hold your face about 10 in (25 cm) above the water, over the scented steam, for 5 minutes. If you find the heat too uncomfortable, come out from under the towel for a moment and then go back under.

3 After steaming, soak a piece of cotton in rosewater (available from drugstores) and gently glide it over your skin to remove any traces of dirt that may have loosened in your pores. As an alternative to rosewater, you can make your own lavender water by infusing a handful of dried lavender in 1 cup (300 ml) of boiling water and letting it cool. Liquidized cucumber is another quick alternative. Moisturize as usual. Please note that steaming your face is not recommended if you have thread veins or very sensitive skin.

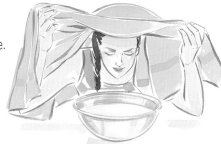

CLEANSE, EXFOLIATE, SOFTEN

■ Regular cleansing, gentle toning, and the use of a light moisturizer night and morning are generally all you need to keep normal skin looking good. However, you may have to adjust this regime in very hot or cold weather—see the tips on the right.

■ To keep normal skin looking fresh and glowing, exfoliate once a week. Skin is constantly growing—making new cells and sloughing off old ones. As you get older this process slows down and can result in a build-up of old cells on the surface of your skin, dulling your complexion. Always choose a gentle exfoliating lotion or, even simpler, gently wipe a wet facecloth in circular motions over the skin.

■ To maximize your naturally clear skin, give yourself a weekly deep-cleansing and softening treatment. To deep-clean your skin, first steam your face as described on the left or use one of the facials on page 112. To nourish and soften it, try the Honey and Orange Softener below. It is a gentle mask, ideal for normal skin.

HONEY AND ORANGE SOFTENER

You will need: *1 tbsp/15 ml honey, few drops of fresh orange juice*

Mix well and spread over cleansed face, avoiding the delicate eye area. Leave on for about 10 minutes. Remove with cotton moistened in warm water.

HELPFUL HEALTH TIPS

■ Use an alcohol-free toner on normal skin. Alcohol is too drying and can irritate skin.

■ Winter weather can strip the skin of its natural oily protection so, even if you normally use soap and water during the rest of the year, switch to a cleansing lotion in cold weather. Use a homemade cleanser, such as milk, olive oil, or sweet almond oil on cotton and wipe gently over the skin.

■ Lack of humidity in heated and air-conditioned offices and houses may mean you have to switch to a heavier moisturizer to compensate.

■ Normal skin can be prone to dryness as you grow older. To combat this, remember to moisturize morning and evening, and have a weekly nourishing treatment. Try the Dry Skin Treat facial oil on page 106. Avoid using the oil around the eyes as it could irritate the thin skin, causing puffiness.

DrySkinCare

Dry skin feels taut after washing and is prone to flakiness. Those with dry skin also tend to have small, almost invisible, pores. Some people suffer from dry skin all their lives; for others it can be due to a seasonal change, lifestyle change, or part of the normal aging process. To keep dry skin looking its best, you need gentle cleansing, regular stimulation with massage, and generous quantities of oil and moisture. If you have some areas of oily skin and some dry areas, use two appropriate cleansers and moisturizers.

DRY SKIN TREAT

You will need: *2 tbsp/30 ml avocado oil, 2 tbsp/30 ml peach-nut or apricot kernel oil, 2 tsp/10 ml wheat germ oil, 10 drops sandalwood essential oil, 5 drops geranium essential oil, 5 drops rose essential oil*

1 Blend the ingredients together and massage the mixture into your face. If you have time, do the facial massage on page 111.

2 Wipe off any excess oil. Any remaining massage oil can be stored in an air-tight container for up to 3 months. Keep it in a dark place.

CLEANSE, EXFOLIATE, MOISTURIZE

■ If a cleanser leaves your skin feeling tight, it is not right for your skin. The alkaline residue left by many soaps can cause this tightening, so if you use soap try changing to a soapfree cleansing bar. Creamy cleansers are better suited to dry skin, but whatever cleanser you use, only cleanse in the evening to get rid of makeup and grime. In the morning, splash your face with warm water or wipe with a facecloth.

■ As skin ages, cell turnover is slowed down. It can be helpful to speed up the process by exfoliating to slough off the dead skin cells that can make skin look sallow and dull. Care should be taken; abrasive exfoliating products can make dry skin drier—causing it to get red and irritated. For a gentler alternative use a soft facecloth (cotton cheesecloth if possible) and massage it gently over the face in circular motions. This will remove dead skin cells without scratching.

■ For an instant nighttime facial oil, pierce either an evening primrose oil capsule or a vitamin E capsule and massage the oil into your skin, avoiding the eye area. If you find this too oily, combine the oil with your usual moisturizer to lighten the mixture.

HELPFUL HEALTH TIPS

■ Avoid toners or skin fresheners that contain alcohol. These remove skin oils that act as natural moisturizers.

■ Light facecloths are available in cosmetic stores and good department stores, but you can make your own by buying a length of plain cotton cheesecloth and cutting it into small squares. Rinse the cloths after every use and put them in the washing machine or boil them every week to remove any bacteria.

■ Avocado pulp or homemade mayonnaise make effective moisturizers for dry skin. Use a thin layer of either as a moisturizer or a thick layer as a hydrating mask.

■ Moisturize dry skin with vitamin-A-rich margarine. A top model swears by it for her beautiful skin. Many women say rubbing margarine on their stomach helps prevent stretch marks during pregnancy.

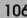

OilySkinCare

f your skin is oily and shiny when you wake up in the morning and becomes shiny very quickly after applying makeup, you probably have oily or combination skin. The latter is dry around the cheeks and oily on forehead, nose, and chin.

FACE MASKS FOR OILY SKIN

■ Plain yogurt is used as a face mask in many Eastern countries and is good for oily or combination skins. Cleansing and nourishing, yogurt contains a form of lactic acid, which is a natural but non-abrasive exfoliant, similar to the fruit acids used in many commercial products. Simply massage over your cleansed face, leave on for 10 minutes and rinse off. Apply moisturizer as usual.

■ Mashed strawberries counteract oiliness. Apply to your face as a simple mask. Leave on for 10 minutes and rinse off.

■ Egg white has a tightening and drying effect on oily skin. Whisk and apply or try the egg and vitamin C mask on page 112.

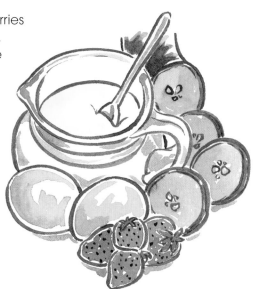

CLEANSE, TONE, MOISTURIZE

■ Oily skin needs to be cleansed twice a day, in the morning and evening, to remove all oil and dirt.

■ It is often claimed that those with oily skins need astringents to help dry up excess oil. This is not true and, in some cases, toners and astringents containing alcohol can actually exacerbate oily skin by drying it out and causing the skin to produce more oil to compensate. Try putting a cucumber in the blender and using the juice as a gentle but effective toner.

■ Oily skin does need moisturizing. Look for moisturizing products that are oil-free and "non comedogenic," which means they will not block the skin's pores and cause pimples. Apply moisturizer around your eyes, the edges of your cheeks (but not the cheekbones), and the neck. Avoid the chin area and the nose; the skin there will produce enough natural lubrication by itself. Adding more can cause enlarged or blocked pores. For combination skin, apply moisturizer to dry areas, but leave oily parts of the face moisture-free.

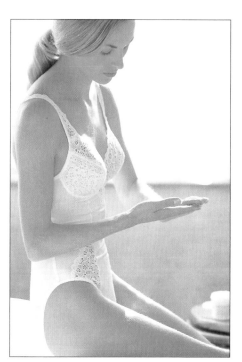

HELPFUL HEALTH TIPS

■ Avoid powdering your face too many times during the day to reduce shine. Layering on powder can form a hard "crust" with oil and sweat, which can lead to blackheads or pimples.

■ If you are buying a face mask for oily skin, choose one containing kaolin or bentonite (clays that help absorb oil), eucalyptus (an oil that draws out impurities), or aluminum magnesium silicate (talc to absorb excess oil).

■ Oily skin is more prone to acne and pimples. If a blemish is on its way, treat it with one of the on-the-spot solutions in Pimple Attack on page 108.

Pimple Attack

Stress, fluctuating hormones, lack of sleep, illness, a reaction to facial products—these can all cause pimples even in those with the most flawless complexions. The trouble starts when the sebaceous glands become disturbed and irritated, which causes redness. The sebum thickens and can become mixed with grime and the debris of dead skin cells blocking the mouth of the pore. Bacteria start to multiply, and a pimple soon appears. Here are some natural solutions that take a matter of minutes.

STRAIGHT TO THE SPOT

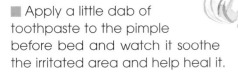

■ Dab a little lemon juice or vitamin C powder on at night and by morning the pimple should have improved. The vitamin C in lemon juice is well known for its healing properties.

■ Apply a little dab of toothpaste to the pimple before bed and watch it soothe the irritated area and help heal it.

■ Apply a drop of undiluted lavender oil or tea tree oil to the pimple. All essential oils have antiseptic properties to varying degrees, but these two are particularly effective for pimples. It is unusual to use essential oils undiluted on the skin, but a tiny drop of either of these two oils will help the blemish to heal more quickly.

BLEMISH MASSAGE OIL

You will need: *3 tbsp/45 ml jojoba oil, 10 drops essential lavender oil, 10 drops essential tea tree oil*

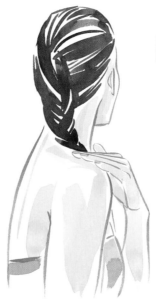

1 Pimples can occur wherever the sebaceous glands are most active. This includes the back, chest, and even the shoulders. Try this simple massage oil to help clear up blemished areas. Blend the oils together and massage gently into any problem areas on shoulders, back, or chest.

2 Ask a friend or partner to rub the massage oil into areas that are hard to reach.

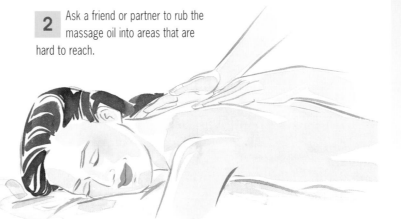

HELPFUL HEALTH TIPS

■ Never squeeze pimples. You run the risk of permanently scarring the skin. Try some of the Straight to the Spot treatments listed here and be patient. If you have a big event to go to, use some concealer or a cover-up stick as a quick fix.

■ The link between eating junk food and getting pimples is largely unproven, but it makes sense to eat a balanced diet high in skin-enhancing vitamins (particularly A, C, and E) and drink plenty of water to detox your body.

■ If you get a sudden and unexpected pimple breakout in your thirties or forties after having years of perfectly clear skin, change your skincare products and treat your skin gently. Do not scrub or exfoliate, causing unnecessary irritation. Try the essential oils suggested on this page, but if there is no improvement see your doctor.

LookingAfterEyes

Your eyes are constantly on show and quickly reveal signs of stress, tiredness, ill health, sun damage, or over-indulgence in alcohol. The skin around the eye is thin and delicate and, unsurprisingly, is one of the first places to develop lines and wrinkles. The skin here also has a tendency to be drier because oil glands in the eye area are fewer and smaller than in other parts of the face. For these reasons your eyes need special care and attention to avoid problems such as dark circles and puffiness.

ONE-MINUTE EYE MASSAGE

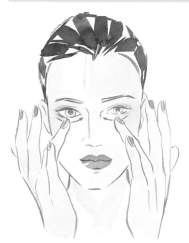 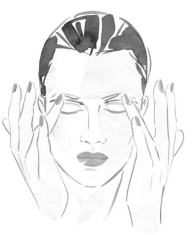

1 Run your hands under cool water. Then, working slowly from the outer corner of the eye to the inner corner, lightly "tap" under the eye for 30 seconds using your ring fingers.

2 Working slowly from the outer corner of the eye to the inner corner, gently tap above the eyes, over the brow bone and the socket area, for another 30 seconds.

HELP FOR PUFFY EYES

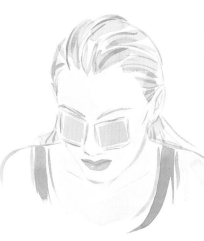

To reduce puffiness, lie down and place cool, moist teabags over your eyes. Pat a thin layer of moisturizer around the eyes before applying the teabags to stop the tea from staining the skin. Relax for 10 minutes. Take the opportunity to do the Rest and Restore Routine on page 98.

OTHER EYE SOLUTIONS

■ Vigorous exercise stimulates lymph drainage, which helps to reduce puffiness around eyes. Cutting down on salt and alcohol should also help the problem.

■ Place chilled slices of cucumber, apple, or potato over tired eyes for 10 minutes to refresh them.

■ To refresh bloodshot, tired eyes, simply splash with ice-cold water when you get up in the morning.

■ Wrap some grated cucumber in cheesecloth and place over eyes for 10 minutes to reduce dark circles.

■ Use raw egg white to tighten skin under the eyes. Simply paint on the whisked egg white 10 minutes before applying your makeup.

■ Don't peer through smeary glasses. Keep them clean.

TIPS
HELPFUL HEALTH

■ Staring at a computer screen all day can cause eyestrain and redness. Take regular breaks from your screen—a couple of minutes every hour if you can. Alter the focus of your eyes from the screen to distant objects at regular intervals.

■ If you are generally healthy, exercise, drink plenty of water, keep to a low-salt diet, sleep well, and still get puffy eyes in the morning, you could be allergic to a beauty product you are using. Try to isolate the culprit, whether it's eye makeup, eye makeup remover, contact lens solution, skincare product—by stopping use one at a time.

■ To help keep eyelashes lustrous and strong, wash an old mascara wand and brush a little jojoba oil on your eyelashes before you go to bed at night.

■ Use almond oil as a gentle eye makeup remover.

Neck Care

The neck has only a small number of fat cells and scant supplies of sebum—the skin's natural oil. This makes the area prone to dryness. The neck is also a prime site of tension. This is not surprising when you consider that it has to support a 10-pound (over 4 kg) weight—your head—all day!

FOR A TENSE NECK

1 Place the middle three fingers of each hand behind your ears, just below the area where you can feel the two round knobbly bones.

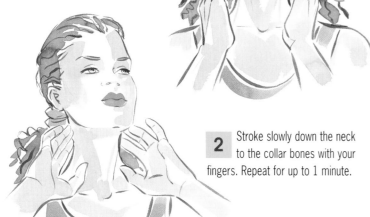

2 Stroke slowly down the neck to the collar bones with your fingers. Repeat for up to 1 minute.

MOISTURIZING

Moisturize your neck twice daily. You may need to use a cream or oil that is richer than the one you use on your face. Work the moisturizer up from the base of your neck all over the neck and behind the ears. Always sweep it in an upward direction to help stop the skin from sagging. Do not forget your neck when you are protecting your skin from the sun. Use plenty of high-factor sun protection and don't forget the area directly under the chin.

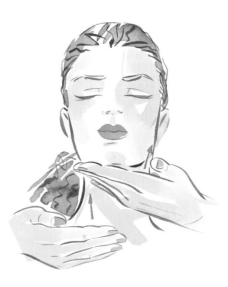

THROAT MASSAGE

Sit upright with your neck straight and place the fingers of one hand on one side of your throat and the thumb on the other. Make quick circular motions up and down the throat. Repeat, using the other hand. You can use a relaxing aromatherapy massage oil during this massage to make it extra effective. Check out Calming Scents on page 88.

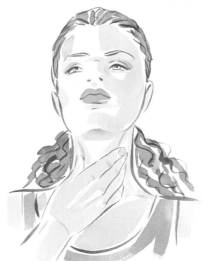

TIPS

■ If you have a short neck, you can give the impression of length by choosing clothes with V-necks or open necks. Avoid fancy collars, or anything that is high or tight around the neck since they will make it look shorter.

■ Sagging muscles can make the jawline heavier, the neck more lined, and the throat muscles sag. Exercise this area with a facial workout. Turn to the Facial Workout on page 42.

■ To extend your neck to its maximum length and improve your posture, imagine a string is attached to the crown of your head. As you sit at your desk or at the dinner table, imagine someone is pulling the string gently upward.

■ The neck is the site of a lot of stress and tension. If you feel stressed, and your neck and shoulders feel stiff and tense, look through Section 4—Calm & Relax for lots of helpful relaxation tips and techniques.

FantasticFastFacial

This very quick and simple massage can help rejuvenate tired, sallow skin and alleviate puffiness and blocked pores by stimulating the lymph nodes. Do it once or twice a week and you should soon see the texture of your skin improve. Before the massage, first cleanse your skin, then use your usual moisturizer as a massage oil. On very dry skins use a little avocado flesh or olive oil.

TEN-MINUTE FACIAL

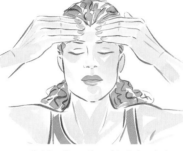

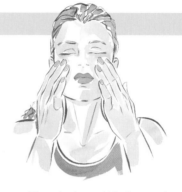

1 Dot moisturizer over your face and neck. Starting behind the ears, use the pads of your fingertips to massage firmly, but slowly, in a circular motion down to the base of your neck. Keep fingertips well lubricated.

2 Put the fingertips of both hands in the middle of your forehead, press firmly, hold for 30 seconds. Release. Move your fingers slightly apart. Repeat. Continue across to the temples.

3 Place the three middle fingers of each hand almost flat against your face at nostril level. Apply pressure, hold, and release. Continue in small steps down toward your jawline.

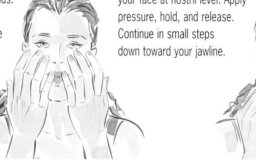

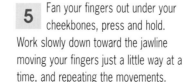

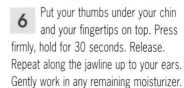

4 Place the pads of your fingertips on your upper lip, press down firmly and hold, then release. Move your fingers to the corners of your mouth and repeat the action.

5 Fan your fingers out under your cheekbones, press and hold. Work slowly down toward the jawline moving your fingers just a little way at a time, and repeating the movements.

6 Put your thumbs under your chin and your fingertips on top. Press firmly, hold for 30 seconds. Release. Repeat along the jawline up to your ears. Gently work in any remaining moisturizer.

HELPFUL HEALTH TIPS

■ The massage facial on this page is not only a great skin rejuvenator, it also helps you to relax. At the end of the facial, close your eyes for a few moments, breathe slowly and deeply, and feel the stress lifting from your face. Unfurrow your brow, unclench your teeth, and "relax" your whole face. Nothing ages your skin more than stress.

■ Exercise is the cheapest way to give your skin a healthy glow and that "just-had-a-facial" look. Section 1—Get Moving! is packed with ideas. Try the warm-up routine on page 12. It's great for energizing you and improving your circulation.

■ The Ten-minute Facial can also be performed with the Aftersun Oil on page 113 if you have been out in the sun all day.

Ten-minute Masks

A weekly face mask can help to improve blood circulation, deep cleanse your skin, or add extra moisture, all depending on the mask you use. Skin products containing vitamin C are big in the cosmetics industry, and a "serum-style" mask is one of the quickest masks you can create, at minimum expense, for an instant beauty boost.

AVOCADO MASK FOR ALL SKIN TYPES

You will need: *1 ripe avocado*

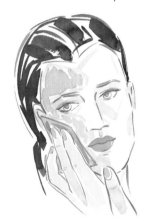
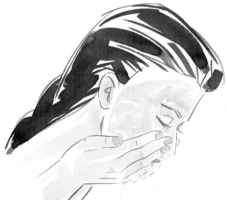

1 Cut open the avocado and scoop out most of the flesh, leaving a little on the skins. Put the flesh to one side to use for other beauty treatments. Cleanse your face. Rub the skins gently over your face, leaving a thin layer of the flesh behind.

2 Relax for 10 minutes. Take the opportunity to check out the visualization exercise on page 86 or the Rest and Restore Routine on page 98. Rinse off the avocado flesh with warm water and lightly pat dry. Moisturize the skin while damp.

"SERUM" MASK FOR ALL SKIN TYPES

You will need: *1 egg white, 1 tsp/5 ml vitamin C powder*

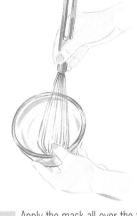

1 Whisk the egg white with the vitamin C powder. If the powder you have bought is a little coarse, chop it finer using a small, sharp knife.

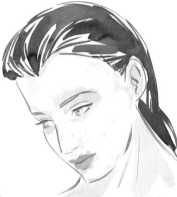

2 Apply the mask all over the face and neck, avoiding the eye area. Leave on for 10 minutes and rinse off with warm or tepid water. Lightly pat your face dry and moisturize.

■ For other beneficial egg-based masks, simply replace the vitamin C in this recipe, with one of these alternatives: 1 teaspoon (5 ml) skimmed milk powder to soften skin; 1 teaspoon (5 ml) honey to moisturize; 1 tablespoon (15 ml) lemon juice for oily skin; 2 tablespoons (30 ml) chopped fresh herbs for oily skin; or 1 egg yolk and 2 tablespoons (30 ml) milk to help combat wrinkles.

CITRUS MASK FOR OILY SKINS

You will need: *2 tsp/10 ml lemon juice, 1 tsp/5 ml lime juice, 1 tsp/5 ml orange juice, 1 carton plain yogurt*

Mix all the ingredients in a bowl. Spread the mixture gently over the face, leave for 10 minutes, and rinse off with warm water.

HELPFUL HEALTH TIPS

■ Raid the fruit bowl for some instant face-mask ideas. Spread mashed bananas over your face, relax for 10 minutes, and rinse off. Bananas are a good moisturizer for dry skins. A mashed pineapple mask exfoliates and will leave your skin smooth and soft. Purée some cucumber to make a soothing mask for sunburn. A mask that will suit either an oily or a combination skin is mashed strawberries!

■ Carrots are high in betacarotene, which is converted by the body into vitamin A—great for cell regeneration. Try this carrot facial for all skin types. Grate 2 carrots, add 1 teaspoon (5 ml) rosewater. Apply to cleansed skin, leave for 10 minutes, and rinse with warm water.

■ If you have a combination skin (some parts are oily and some are dry), use two suitable face masks on the different areas.

SaferSuncare

The sun has had a very bad press over the past few years. The aging effects caused by sun damage are well documented, and the incidence of skin cancer is on the increase. While the sun undoubtedly damages the skin, it also makes most people feel good and more relaxed—it has been shown to lower blood pressure. So the message is—enjoy the sun, but do so as safely as possible.

TEN SUNNING ESSENTIALS

1 Even if there is cloud cover when you go outdoors you should use a sunscreen.

2 Make sure the sunscreen you choose protects you from UVA and UVB rays.

3 White skins shouldn't use anything lower than a Sun Protection Factor (SPF)15–20. Very pale skin types, babies, young children, and those who want complete sun protection should opt for SPF 30.

Take Care

The sun's ultraviolet UVA rays speed up signs of aging, damage the skin's elasticity, and increase the long-term risk of skin cancer. UVB rays cause sunburn and redness and some types of cancer.

4 Never sunbathe under the midday sun. The sun is at its hottest, and most damaging, between 11 a.m. and 3 p.m., so stay in the shade or cover up during this time.

5 Many cosmetics come with a built-in sunscreen and can help to protect the skin on a daily basis, but if you are out in hot sun, you will need a high-protection sunscreen.

6 Apply sunscreen regularly and liberally when you are in the sun. If you go into the water and towel dry afterward, reapply your sunscreen, even if it is labeled "waterproof."

7 Don't rub your sunscreen in too hard—being over-enthusiastic with the lotion can reduce its efficiency by about 25 percent. Sunscreen does not last forever—check the "use-by" date on old bottles and throw away out-of-date lotions.

8 Apply a thorough layer of sunscreen to your naked body before going out into the sun. That way, you won't miss areas around the straps of your swimsuit. Remember to pay special attention to bony areas such as the top of the feet, neck bones, and nose.

9 If you suddenly run out of sunscreen, you can try your kitchen cupboard for a simple solution—sesame oil! This oil offers a little protection from UV rays, but purchased sunscreens offer much more effective protection.

10 Spread a layer of blended cucumber, strawberries, or tomatoes over sunburned skin.

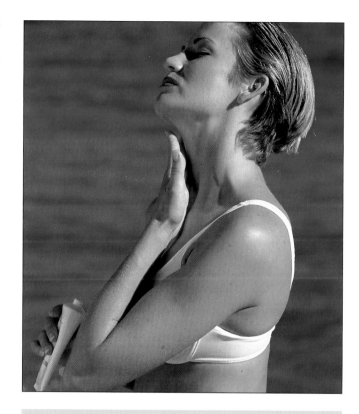

AFTERSUN OIL

You will need: *1 tbsp/15 ml wheat germ oil, 2 tbsp/30 ml grapeseed oil, 2 tbsp/30 ml olive oil, 10 drops chamomile essential oil, 5 drops bergamot essential oil, 5 drops myrrh essential oil*

Mix all the ingredients together. Apply to sun-damaged skin. The high vitamin E content in this mixture cannot undo years of sun damage, but can help to minimize further damage.

HairConditioningTreatments

Hair is an excellent barometer of your health. If you are ill, stressed, tired, or not eating properly, your hair will not be at its best. The main requirement for healthy, shiny hair is taking care of yourself. Check out the other sections in this book for advice on exercise, healthy eating, and reducing stress. Taking care of your hair on a regular basis will also help keep it looking good. The treatments described here, and on the following pages, use readily available ingredients and will also help to improve the condition of your scalp.

AVOCADO DRY HAIR SAVER

You will need: ½ avocado, 3 tbsp/45 ml olive oil

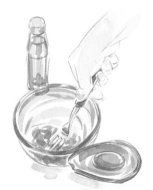 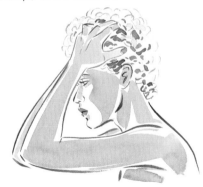

1 Scoop out the avocado flesh and mash it. Add the olive oil and blend with the avocado.

2 Massage into dry hair. If your scalp is oily, put the mixture on the ends only. Wrap a towel around your hair and leave for 10 minutes. Shampoo and rinse.

OILY HAIR

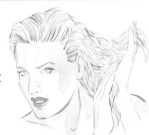

Opinion is divided over whether oily hair needs conditioning since there is already a lot of oil in it. Some people believe that adding more moisturizer can make it lanker and greasier. The answer is to coat only the ends of the hair with conditioner (to prevent them from becoming split and dry), avoiding the scalp completely. Rinse off the conditioner thoroughly.

QUICK CONDITIONERS

■ Massage mayonnaise into dry hair. If your scalp is oily, coat the hair-ends only. Wrap hair in a warm towel and leave for 10 minutes. Shampoo and rinse.

■ Eggs are renowned for making hair shine. To make your own egg treatment, crack two eggs into a bowl. Add 2 tablespoons (30 ml) of olive oil to the eggs and mix. First shampoo your hair as usual and towel dry. Massage in the egg mixture and leave for 10 minutes. Rinse well.

■ For an intensive hair-conditioning treatment, warm 2 tablespoons (30 ml) olive oil and massage into the hair. If your scalp is oily, coat the ends only. Wrap a warm towel or plastic wrap around your hair and relax for 10 minutes.

■ To treat dandruff, try this simple scalp massage. Mix 3 tablespoons (45 ml) jojoba oil with 20 drops of tea tree oil. Decant into a container. Massage a small amount of the oil into the scalp with your fingertips using firm circular movements. Shampoo and rinse. Use 2 or 3 times a week.

HELPFUL HEALTH TIPS

■ Sun, salt water, and chlorine can all have disastrous effects on the color and condition of your hair. Wear a hat to protect your hair from the sun and look out for hair sprays and protectors containing UV filters.

■ Your hair can become oilier due to changes in hormone levels in the body—before your period, during pregnancy, and during menopause. At these times you may find you have to change your hair-care routine and wash your hair more than usual. Do not exacerbate the problem of oiliness by using conditioner on your scalp.

■ Some scalp conditions seem to be aggravated by eating dairy products. If you suffer badly from dandruff, try cutting dairy products out of your diet for 2–4 weeks to see if the condition improves. If it doesn't, ask your doctor to refer you to a dermatologist.

Rinse&Shine

Hair rinses are an easy step towards healthier hair. They should be used as the last step in a hair-care routine, helping to add shine and often a wonderful perfume. Natural hair rinses and tonics can be prepared in a matter of minutes and are easy to use. The shine-enhancing suggestions listed here require ingredients that you probably already have in your kitchen or bathroom.

TEN RINSES IN MINUTES

1 Raspberry rinse for oily hair
Try this raspberry rinse to give shine to oily hair. Extract the juice from 4 oz (125 g) raspberries by pushing them through a strainer or using a juicer. Combine the juice with 1 teaspoon (5 ml) honey, ½ teaspoon (2.5 ml) crushed cloves, and 1 quart (1 liter) distilled vinegar. Decant the mixture into a bottle. Shake well. Dilute one part to six parts water and keep the remainder in the fridge. Use as a final rinse after shampooing and conditioning.

2 Mint shine for greasy hair
Infuse 2 mint teabags in a quart (1 liter) of boiling bottled water for about 10 minutes. After shampooing and conditioning, pour the warm mint tea over your hair for shine without greasiness.

3 Fragrant rinse
All hair types will benefit from this. Add 5 drops rose essential oil to 1 quart (1 liter) bottled water and shake well. Use as a rinse after shampooing.

4 To make dull hair shine
Mix together 1 cup (250 ml) white wine vinegar and 1 quart (1 liter) boiling water. Let it cool slightly. Work into shampooed and conditioned hair, then rinse off with iced water.

5 To make dark hair shine
To make dark hair shine, add 5 drops rosemary essential oil to 1 quart (1 liter) bottled water, shake well, and use as a final rinse.

6 To make blond hair shine
Add 5 drops chamomile essential oil to 1 quart (1 liter) bottled water, shake well. Use as a final rinse. If you have time and want a more concentrated highlighter, infuse 4 tablespoons (60 ml) dried chamomile flowers in ½ cup (125 ml) boiling water for 10–20 minutes. Strain and apply the liquid to shampooed, wet hair. Leave the infusion on for 20 minutes, then rinse out.

7 Herb rinses
Herbs and herbal teabags can be used to combat dry or oily hair conditions and to add shine. Make an infusion with 4 tablespoons (60 ml) dried herbs or 2 herbal teabags to 1 quart (1 liter) boiling water. When lukewarm, rub the rinse into your hair after shampooing.

For oily hair choose lavender, lemon balm, rosemary, thyme, or yarrow. Dry hair will benefit from a final rinse of comfrey, parsley, or sage. To keep normal hair healthy, treat it gently with sage, chamomile, elderflower, or geranium.

8 Anti-dandruff
Mix together 1 cup (250 ml) mouthwash with 1 cup (250 ml) witchhazel and decant the solution into a spray-topped container. Shampoo and condition your hair as usual. Towel dry and spritz the mixture onto your scalp.

9 Chlorine cure
If disaster strikes and your over-lightened, or bleached, hair takes on a tinge of green after contact with chlorinated water, try this rinse with a difference! Massage a few tablespoons of tomato ketchup into your hair and leave for 10–30 minutes. Rinse out thoroughly.

10 Oil reducer
For oily hair, put 2 teaspoons of lemon juice in a jug of cold water and use for a final rinse after shampooing.

Smart**Hands**

Many of us invest a lot of time in looking after the skin on our faces, but forget about the skin on our hands. The result? Your face may appear years younger than you actually are, but your hands will give the game away. The solution? Invest a little bit of time caring for your hands.

LUXURY HAND OIL

You will need: 3 tbsp/45 ml jojoba oil, 3 tbsp/ 45 ml sesame or almond oil, 10 drops sandalwood and rose essential oils

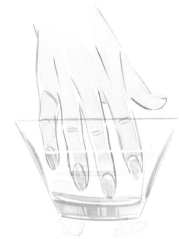

Mix all the ingredients together and pour into a bottle. Massage a few drops into your hands daily, particularly after you have had your hands in water. Sesame and almond oil are also mild natural sunscreens, so this hand oil will give your hands some protection from UV rays.

HAND SHAKE AND STRETCH

Exercising your hands often can help prevent conditions like repetitive strain injury and stiff, arthritic joints. It also helps to tone up the skin on the hands, which tends to become looser as we age. Shake your hands loosely from the wrists, letting your fingers flap together. Then fan out your fingers as far as they will go. Hold for 5 seconds, then release. Move your fingers as if you are playing an imaginary piano. Try this routine a couple of times a day.

1 To strengthen your nails, soak them in 4 tablespoons (60 ml) cider vinegar for 2 minutes. Alternatively, put 1 teaspoon (5 ml) table salt in a glass of cold water and soak your nails in the solution for 2 minutes.

2 File nails with an emery board in one direction only. Do not use a metal file, which can damage the nail. Avoid shaping nails too much at the sides, which causes them to break. Keep your finger nails neat and short—especially if they are brittle or damaged. Trying to grow them when they are weak makes them more likely to catch on something. They are easier to look after when they are short.

3 If you paint your nails, always wear a base coat under the polish to stop staining. Bear in mind that it is better to touch up nail polish if it becomes chipped than to remove it. Peeling off polish or using polish remover frequently can weaken nails.

4 To dry nail polish in a hurry, use a hair dryer on a low, cool setting. Hold the dryer 12 in (30 cm) away and blow air over your nails for 20 seconds. Alternatively, dip your nails in a bowl of ice water.

HELPFUL HEALTH **TIPS**

■ For an intensive, overnight hand treatment, massage one tablespoon (15 ml) of the Luxury Hand Oil or other good emollient hand cream into your hands, nails, and cuticles. Then put on a pair of cotton gloves and wear them overnight.

■ To improve the condition of the skin on your hands, buy unperfumed dishwashing detergent and add a few drops of your favorite essential oil to the water. Lemon is lovely and fresh, as is peppermint. The oils are also antiseptic and perfectly hygienic to use on your cleaning cloths and all kitchen surfaces.

■ Prevent brown liver spots on your hands by protecting them from the sun with a high-factor sun protection cream (15+). Gently "bleach" any liver spots by soaking your hands in the juice of 1 lemon mixed with 2 teaspoons (10 ml) olive oil for 10 minutes.

■ There are more hand exercises to try on page 95.

TreatsForFeet

Every time you take a step, your feet absorb the stress of up to twice your body weight—and even more when you are running or jumping. In a lifetime your feet carry you thousands of miles. They may not be on show much, except in the summer, but your feet do deserve a bit of tender loving care. Here are some quick toe tips!

FIZZY FOOT SPA

You will need: 2 drops each lemon and lime essential oils, 3 tbsp/45 ml sodium bicarbonate or baking soda, 1 tbsp/15 ml citric acid

Dissolve all the ingredients in a large bowl of hot water and soak your feet for 10 minutes— or as long as you want.

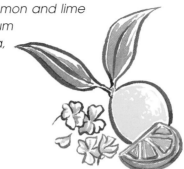

TEN-MINUTE PEDICURE

You will need: essential oils (lavender or peppermint), pumice stone, oatmeal, (or sea salt and olive oil), almond oil

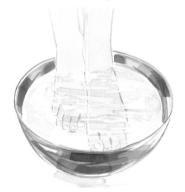 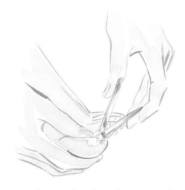 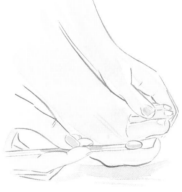 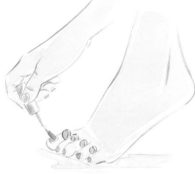

1 Add a couple of drops of essential oil to a bowl of lukewarm water. Lavender is relaxing and healing; peppermint is cooling for hot, over-tired feet. Soak your feet. After 3–4 minutes, slough off the dead skin with a pumice stone or exfoliant, such as a handful of oatmeal or olive oil and coarse sea salt.

2 Remove feet from the water and dry them thoroughly. Cut your toenails straight across. Curved toenails can lead to in-growing toenails.

3 Massage your feet with a mixture of a little almond oil and peppermint or lavender essential oil. Use sweeping movements to massage from the toes to the ankles. Rub oil into the cuticle area and push back cuticles with a cotton swab, or orange stick.

4 If you are going to polish your nails, wash them in warm soapy water to remove the oil before applying the polish. Separate your toes with rolled-up tissues or cotton balls. Apply a base coat to avoid staining nails.

HELPFUL HEALTH TIPS

■ You don't have to save face masks for your face. Use a mask on your feet (see Ten-minute Masks on page 112) to keep the skin of your feet soft and supple. Add eucalyptus or tea tree oil if your feet are sweaty or prone to athlete's foot.

■ To soften hard skin on the feet, add 1 teaspoon (5 ml) malt vinegar to a small container of plain yogurt and rub the mixture all over the hard skin areas. Put your feet up for 5 minutes. Try the Leg and Back Relaxer on page 99. Rinse off the mixture before exfoliating as described in Step 1 on the left.

■ The foot, particularly the sole, contains thousands of nerve endings, and massaging them can stimulate the whole body. Check out the foot massage information on page 92.

■ The feet and toes benefit from exercise—especially after being squashed into shoes all day or walked on for miles! Do the exercises on page 95 to de-stress your feet.

Body Care

It takes only a few minutes a day to keep your skin looking good from head to toe, and regular attention will result in a smooth, soft, younger-looking body for life. Try this skin-smoothing routine once or twice a week. Milk will soften the skin and loosen dead skin cells. Gentle exfoliation with oatmeal or salt will bring a glow back to dull-looking skin. The ingredients used here are inexpensive and readily available.

TEN MINUTES TO SOFT SKIN

You will need to cleanse and exfoliate: 2 cups/1 pint/600 ml whole milk or 1 cup/250 g powdered milk, a few drops almond or olive oil, a handful of sea salt or coarsely ground oatmeal
To moisturize: olive or almond oil, or vitamin E or evening primrose oil capsules, or moisturizing body lotion

1 To give your body a deep cleansing and exfoliating treatment in the bath, first add the milk and oil to a bathful of warm water. Soak in the milky water for 5 minutes. (Milk contains naturally occurring alpha hydroxy acids (AHAs). Synthetically produced versions of AHAs are found in many purchased anti-aging skincare products.) Stand up in the tub. Take care, as the milky water may make the tub slippery. Put the salt or oatmeal on a washcloth and gently massage the skin to rub off dead skin cells.

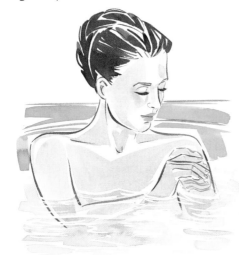

2 Shower off the oatmeal or salt with warm water, then give your body a final blast with cold water. Cold water is not only refreshing, it should help to stimulate and tone your skin. If you want your breasts to stay firm, spray them each morning with a blast of cold water.

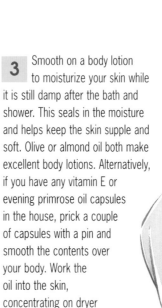

3 Smooth on a body lotion to moisturize your skin while it is still damp after the bath and shower. This seals in the moisture and helps keep the skin supple and soft. Olive or almond oil both make excellent body lotions. Alternatively, if you have any vitamin E or evening primrose oil capsules in the house, prick a couple of capsules with a pin and smooth the contents over your body. Work the oil into the skin, concentrating on dryer areas such as shins, elbows, and knees.

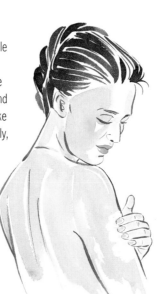

HELPFUL HEALTH TIPS

■ For best results when exfoliating, massage using circular movements, concentrating on areas such as knees, elbows, feet, and backs of thighs.

■ Exfoliation improves skin tone and provides a good base for applying a fake tan. If you don't exfoliate, the tan will stick to the dry, flaky skin and make the "tan" appear patchy. Exfoliation before sunbathing helps you get a more even natural tan, too.

■ Pimples can occur anywhere on the body where there is a high concentration of sebaceous glands. Problem areas include the shoulders, chest, and back. Treat pimples gently with the remedies suggested in Pimple Attack on page 108.

■ Cut a lemon in half and squeeze out the juice. (You can use the juice as a hair rinse if you have oily hair—see page 115). Rest your elbows in the lemon skins for 5–10 minutes. This has a gently bleaching effect, and the fruit acids exfoliate cracked, dry skin.

WarOnCellulite

Cellulite, the dimpled, spongy flesh caused by swollen fat cells, is the bane of many women's lives. Poor circulation, hormonal changes, food allergies, and environmental toxins have all been blamed. But whatever the cause, the condition can be vastly improved by taking just a few minutes a day to increase your circulation and improve lymphatic drainage (your lymph glands, situated in the neck, under the arms, and in the groin, help to rid the body of toxins). Skin brushing improves lymphatic drainage. A salt rub is particularly effective on problem areas. Anti-cellulite oil works by increasing circulation and eliminating toxins. Choose any one of these three treatments if time is short. Combine them for a really effective "war on cellulite" when time allows.

BODY BRUSHING

Using a long-handled natural bristle brush, simply brush your skin before you get in the bath or shower. Start at the feet and brush your skin in firm, sweeping upward movements. Brush firmly enough to produce a pink glow on the skin. Brush the whole of your body in this way, paying particular attention to cellulite-prone areas. Aim to do this daily. It will improve your skin tone and is one of the simplest, most effective, treatments in helping to disperse the fatty deposits that may cause cellulite.

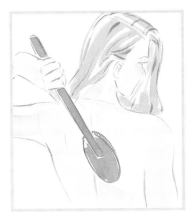

ANTI-CELLULITE RUB

You will need: a handful of coarse sea salt mixed with 1 tbsp/15 ml olive oil

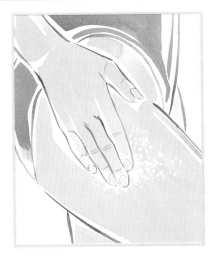

Rub the mixture of sea salt and olive oil into areas affected by cellulite on your body. Rinse off well in the bath or shower.

ANTI-CELLULITE OIL

You will need: 1 tsp/5 ml wheat germ oil, 3 tbsp/ 45 ml grapeseed oil, 10 drops juniper essential oil, 10 drops lemon essential oil, 5 drops cypress essential oil

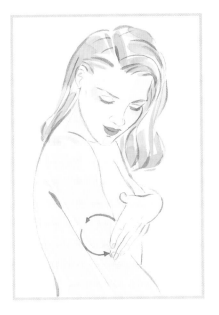

Blend the oils together. Massage the mixture into cellulite-prone regions (hips, buttocks, inner thighs, upper arms), using firm, circular motions. For extra effectiveness, use after body brushing and after the anti-cellulite salt rub.

HELPFUL HEALTH TIPS

■ The essential oils used in the Anti-cellulite Oil described here can also be added to your bath to help combat cellulite. Mix with a carrier oil first—see Calming Scents on page 88.

■ To help eliminate or prevent cellulite, you need to think about your body on the inside, too. Drink plenty of water and take time to exercise, as cellulite is often a sign that you are storing too much fat.

■ Try to avoid drastic weight changes, which can lead to cellulite. If you are dieting, aim for a steady weight loss of around 2 lb (1 kg) a week.

■ Taking extra estrogen can make cellulite worse. If you take the combined oral contraceptive pill, ask your doctor if it is possible to switch to a lower-dose formulation. Alternatively, switch to the progesterone-only pill or use a barrier method of contraception.

WaterTherapy

I t's free (well, almost) and forms the basis of moisturizers and many beauty treatments. So splash it all over, cleanse with it, drink it, moisturize with it, and for puffy eyes and skin, freeze it and use it. Go water wild!

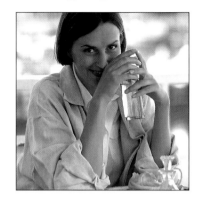

WATER

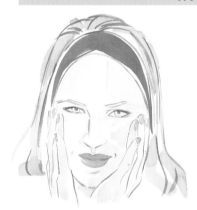
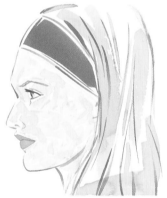

1 To trap moisture, after cleansing (and exfoliating, if necessary) lightly pat your face with a clean towel to remove excess water only. Apply your moisturizer while the skin is damp. This will help to keep your skin soft and supple.

2 Use a face mask to keep moisture in your skin if your skin is very dry—perhaps because you've been out in the wind or sun. Apply a face mask (see Ten-Minute Masks on page 112) over moisturized skin and relax for 10 minutes.

STEAM

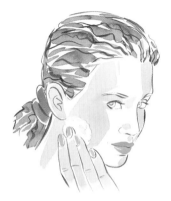
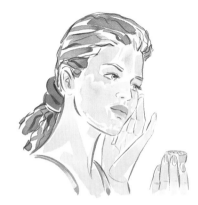

1 Before taking a bath, cleanse your face. Try dipping a ball of cotton in milk and rubbing over the face for an instant cleanser. The steam from your bath water can then help to deep-cleanse your face by causing the skin to perspire. It also helps soften or release sebum that may block pores.

2 Exfoliate in the steamy bathroom after your bath for best results. The enzymes and fruit acids in some exfoliators are activated by steam and will penetrate the skin more effectively. Massage the flesh of a passion fruit, which contains natural fruit acids, gently into the skin. Rinse well. Pat skin dry and moisturize.

ICE

Wrap a pack of frozen peas in a cloth and place over eyes for 5–10 minutes. The chill factor helps diminish bags and "red eye" by constricting the blood vessels. Alternatively, keep two teaspoons in the freezer, and when you need them, wrap them in a cloth and place one teaspoon over each eye. Stainless steel is better than silver, which warms up more quickly.

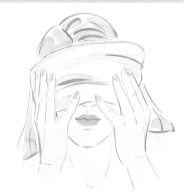

HELPFUL HEALTH TIPS

■ To reduce the dehydrating effects of stuffy centrally heated rooms, place a bowl of water in the room. Add a few drops of your favorite essential oil to enhance your mood.

■ Aim to drink as much water as you can throughout the day (at least six large glasses). This will help to keep your kidneys working, detox your body, and help improve your skin. If you don't drink enough water, your body starts to draw on its water reservoirs (including those of your skin) making skin duller and possibly oilier or drier. If you want to add a little more excitement to your drinking water, freeze some fruit juices in your ice cube tray and add them.

■ Carbonated water is harder to drink in a large volume because the gassiness of the water fills you up. So if you are trying to drink more water, it may be best to stick to plain water.

Shower**Power**

here is no simpler and quicker beauty enhancer than taking a shower. A warm bath can be pleasant for relaxing at the end of a hard day, but a shower offers you more advantages on the beauty front. This is because the spray from the shower has a massaging effect on the skin. Also, because you are standing up, fluids drain from your face, joints, and upper body, helping to reduce puffiness and bloating. A shower is also less drying to the skin than a bath because there is less prolonged contact with water. The shower makes your skin damp, rather than soaking it, which makes it a better place to use exfoliating body scrubs and loofahs.

FOOT SMOOTHIE

Run warm water over your feet to soften the skin. Sit on a shower stool to exfoliate the skin on the soles and sides of your feet. Use circular motions with either a long-handled brush or an exfoliating scrub (see Body Care on page 118). End the treatment with a spray of cold water on the sensitive soles of your feet.

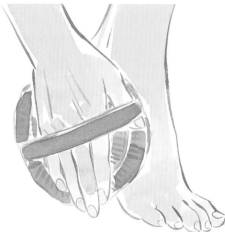

BOOST ENERGY & EXFOLIATE

Alternate between warm and cool water and exfoliate in a circular motion—either with a long-handled brush or an exfoliating scrub (see Body Care on page 118). Start massaging your body from the bottom of your feet and work upward to boost blood circulation and invigorate yourself. Finish off with a final blast of cold water.

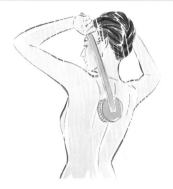

COMBAT A COLD

1 If your sinuses are blocked through over-dry central heating or you have a cold, stand under the shower and let warm water run over your face to drain your nasal passages.

2 Massage the bridge of your nose with your thumbs to help clear your sinuses.

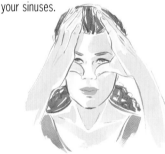

3 To relieve aches and pains, direct the water from the shower onto your calves and let it run for a few minutes before ending with a quick blast of cool water.

4 Finally, add a couple of drops of eucalyptus oil to your sponge or facecloth, rub over the body, and inhale the vapors.

HELPFUL HEALTH **TIPS**

■ Extend your foot massage after the shower by mixing a couple of drops of peppermint and tea tree oils with 1 tablespoon (15 ml) olive oil. Rub gently over the feet.

■ Shower treatments work best in showers that allow you to control the temperature, speed, and spray intensity. There is a range of different shower heads available, and it may be worth investing in a new one.

■ Soothe tight, tired, or swollen muscles at the back of your neck by directing the water flow from your shower onto the problem area. Use the strongest pressure you can get from your shower to massage this all-important stress point.

Blissful**BathSoaks**

Relaxing at the end of the day in a hot, candlelit bath is one of life's luxuries, a great de-stresser, and a prelude to winding down to a good night's sleep. There are plenty of bath foams, salts, and oils available in stores, but many of these contain a great deal of detergent and can be drying to the skin. Making your own bath soaks is not only better for your skin, but also allows you to create personalized treatments to suit your particular mood or the condition of your skin.

MILK AND HONEY BATH

You will need: *1 cup/½ pint/300 ml whole milk or 1 tbsp/15 ml dried milk, 4 tbsp/60 ml honey, 2 cups/1 pint/600 ml boiling water*

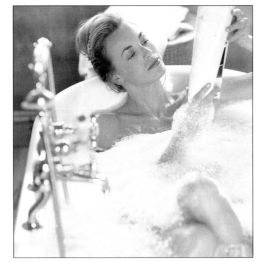

Dissolve the honey in the boiling water and add to the bath. Add the whole milk or dried milk directly under the running water. Lay back in the tub and relax for 10 minutes. The fatty acids in milk, an ancient beautifier, act as an efficient cleanser, and the fat helps prevent the skin from drying out. The honey adds a touch of luxury and will soften the skin.

SPICY WINTER BATH

You will need: *2 cups/1 pint/600 ml rosewater (available from most drugstores), 2 bay leaves, 1 tsp crushed cloves, 2 cups/1 pint/600 ml wine vinegar*

Combine the ingredients and simmer on the stove for 10 minutes or more, adding extra rosewater if the liquid evaporates. Add half a cup to your bath and relax. Store the rest in a cool, dark place and use within one week.

LUXURY ROSE BATH

You will need: *2 tsp/10 ml carrier oil, 2 drops sandalwood essential oil, 5 drops rose essential oil*

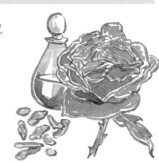

Mix the ingredients together and add to the bath after you have run it. Relax for 10 minutes, inhaling the soothing vapors.

SEXY BATH

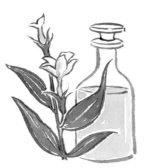

You will need: *2 tsp/10 ml carrier oil, 4 drops patchouli essential oil, 2 drops ylang ylang essential oil, 2 drops jasmine essential oil*

Add the oils to your bath after you have run it, not as the water is running. In this way the heat will not affect the oils, and you can take full advantage of the sensual vapors and supposed aphrodisiac properties! Relax for 10 minutes.

TIPS

HELPFUL HEALTH

■ When taking a scented or aromatherapy bath, close all windows and doors so you get the full fragrance and therapeutic benefits of the oils.

■ Herbal teabags make cheap and relaxing bath soaks. Tie the bag around the faucet in the stream of running water or simply add to a warm bath. Chamomile teabags make relaxing soaks, while lemon and ginger bags have a more revitalizing effect. Berry teas provide a fruit-scented soak.

■ Coconut milk makes a great softening and scented bath soak. Add all the milk from a fresh coconut or 1 tablespoon (15 ml) dried coconut milk powder to your bath.

■ Rose essential oil is a luxurious and uplifting oil that can be used to treat mild fatigue and depression. It can also help ease the symptoms of PMS and menopause.

HomeSpa

Every once in a while, you deserve to forget the clock and turn your home into a spa for a day—or even the weekend. By pulling together many of the 10-minute tips in this book, you can enjoy a day of luxury and look like a million dollars, for just a few cents! Organize your spa day for a time when you can be alone in the house and are relatively free of work or family responsibilities. Do not take work home, ask a family member or friend to take the kids for the day, unplug the telephone, and let people know you do not want to be disturbed. Don't feel guilty about pampering yourself and relaxing. You, and everyone else around you, will benefit if you feel good about yourself.

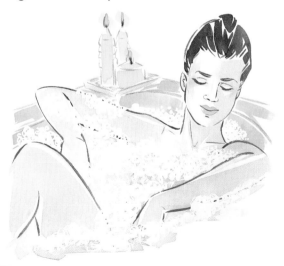

TEN TIPS FOR YOUR HOME SPA

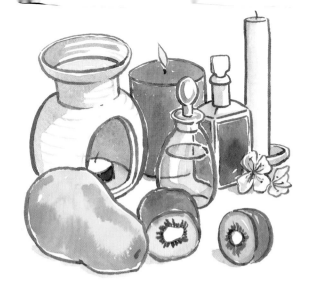

1 Prepare for your day
Stock up on healthy food—preferably fresh fruit and vegetables. Look through Section 3—Eat Well for inspiration. Buy some aromatherapy oils, such as energizing lemon or relaxing geranium, and make your own air-freshener to spray around the house—see Calming Scents on page 88.

2 Start the day well
Begin with a long drink of warm water with a slice of lemon. Aim to drink as much water as you can throughout the day to help flush toxins and hydrate your skin.

3 Cut out caffeine
Avoid coffee and tea and other drinks containing caffeine for the day. Try eating more fruit and drinking mineral water or juices—see pages 58 and 59 for some original ideas for freshly blended fruit and vegetable juices.

4 Beautify that body
Give yourself a facial massage (page 111), a face mask (page 112), and a complete body scrub, tone, and moisturize (page 118).

5 Take it easy
Don't do anything energetic. Take a gentle walk in pleasant surroundings, read a book, or listen to soothing music.

6 Treat your hands and feet
Give yourself a manicure (page 116) and pedicure (page 117).

7 Meditate or visualize
Try meditation (page 90) or the visualization sequence on page 86. It may become a habit!

8 Learn a relaxation technique
If you haven't tried the relaxation routine on page 98—now is the perfect time. If you already use the routine, check through the pages in Section 4—Calm & Relax and try something new.

9 Float your cares away
Dim the lights and light a few candles. Play a relaxing tape. Add one box of Epsom salts to a warm bath. Relax for 15 minutes.

10 Beauty sleep
Skin cells regenerate when you sleep, your face relaxes, wrinkles and lines soften, and you lose that red-eyed, pale-skinned look of the sleep-deprived. Put a few drops of lavender essential oil on your pillow to be sure of a good night's rest.

Body**ActionPlan**

Use this quick guide to target the part of your body you would most like to improve. To exercise, energize, and tone, choose routines from Section 1—Get Moving! and Section 2—Stretch & Tone. To help you relax and de-stress, choose programs from Section 4—Calm & Relax. For skin and hair care, refer to Section 5—Look Good.

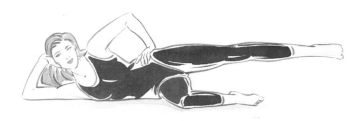

FastFact**Finder**

If you have a particular health or beauty question, use this page to find the ten-minute answer. From losing weight to fighting fatigue—there is something you can do even if you only have minutes to spare. If taking that first step toward a healthier lifestyle is your stumbling block—check out the "Look at the Facts" pages listed below. Choose one that addresses your concerns and leave the easel open on that page. Read it when you need a motivating boost and you'll soon be on your way!

Index

Acknowledgments
Project Editor: Katie Preston
Editors: Stella Vayne and Nicole Foster
Editorial Assistant: Catherine Brereton
Art Director: Robert Mathias
Eat Well recipes: Maggie Mayhew
Exercise illustrations: Catherine Ward/Simon Girling & Associates
Other illustrations: Liz Sawyer/Simon Girling & Associates
Photographs: Tony Stone Images
Cover photographs: PhotoDisc, Inc. and Tony Stone Images

The author wishes to give special thanks to the team at
Tucker Slingsby—Katie, Janet, and Del

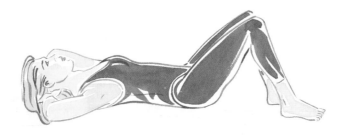